BINAURAL INTERFERENCE

A Guide for Audiologists

Editor-in-Chief for Audiology
Brad A. Stach, PhD

BINAURAL INTERFERENCE

A Guide for Audiologists

James Jerger, PhD
Carol A. Silverman, PhD, MPH

PLURAL PUBLISHING INC.

PLURAL PUBLISHING
INC.

5521 Ruffin Road
San Diego, CA 92123

e-mail: info@pluralpublishing.com
website: http://www.pluralpublishing.com

Typeset in 11/13 Palatino by Flanagan's Publishing Services, Inc.
Printed in the United States of America by McNaughton & Gunn

Library of Congress Cataloging-in-Publication Data

Names: Jerger, James, author. | Silverman, Carol A. (Carol Ann), 1953- author.
Title: Binaural interference : a guide for audiologists / James Jerger, Carol A. Silverman.
Description: San Diego, CA : Plural, [2018] | Includes bibliographical references and index.
Identifiers: LCCN 2017045984 | ISBN 9781635500769 (alk. paper) | ISBN 1635500761 (alk. paper)
Subjects: | MESH: Hearing Loss, Bilateral | Auditory Perceptual Disorders
Classification: LCC RF290 | NLM WV 270 | DDC 617.8—dc23
LC record available at https://lccn.loc.gov/2017045984

Contents

Preface by James Jerger

Many years ago, when I was teaching and researching at the Baylor College of Medicine in Houston, Texas, the public relations people at the medical school arranged for me to be interviewed by a reporter from a local Houston newspaper concerning the research projects we were currently conducting. In the course of the meeting, I mentioned that, while binaural aids were the standard of practice in our audiology clinic, we had identified a few elderly hearing aid users who preferred just one aided ear over both aided ears, and we were trying to understand the basis for this preference. The newspaper published a short piece on this at the bottom of the last column of one of the back pages of the paper. I forgot all about it until weeks later, when I received a short letter from a woman in North Carolina. She asked God to bless me for the item she found in her paper explaining our research. She said that she had been telling her audiologist for months that she didn't do well with both aids on in noisy places. She said that she did much better if she removed the aid from her left ear. Her audiologist had been insisting that she would get used to aids in both ears, but now she was sure that she had been right all along.

Apparently, one of the wire services picked up the item from the Houston paper and it spread nationwide. That single letter from a grateful monaural user convinced me that the apparent interaural conflict generated by binaural fittings in at least some elderly persons warranted serious consideration. I began the study of what came to be called "binaural interference," and have maintained an interest in the phenomenon for almost 50 years. In the 1980s, my good friends and colleagues Shlomo Silman, Carol Silverman, Michele Emmer, and their associates at the City University of New York began a series of studies on the phenomenon of auditory deprivation. It soon became apparent that binaural interference and auditory deprivation were closely related. A research partnership developed between our two labs, resulting in a series of publications based on our joint interests. This book is the result of that long, fruitful, and continuing partnership.

We are indebted to many individuals for assistance with the preparation of this book, but especially Susan Jerger, whose support has been invaluable and unwavering. For their special contribution to our research into binaural interference at the Baylor College of Medicine, thanks to Henry Lew, Rose Chmiel, and Emily Murphy. Thanks, also, to Angie Singh and Valerie Johns, at Plural Publishing, for their much-appreciated support. Finally, we are indebted to Lina Reiss for her generous assistance with the editing of the sections on pitch matching, and for the important contributions that the research of her team at the Oregon Health Science University has made to the study of binaural interference.

—James Jerger, PhD

Preface by Carol A. Silverman

The first study on binaural interference, which resulted from a collaboration between Jim Jerger and his colleagues at Baylor College of Medicine and Shlomo Silman at the Brooklyn College Center for Auditory Research, published about 25 years ago, demonstrated that some individuals, particularly older individuals, perform more poorly with two hearing aids than with one and/or more poorly with binaural than monaural stimulation. Surprisingly, however, given the adverse impact of binaural interference on auditory function, and its occurrence in a significant subset of the population with hearing loss, research on binaural interference only recently has begun to flourish; and adaptation of audiologic clinical practice to identify, assess, and manage individuals with binaural interference has yet to become widespread.

My interest in binaural interference stems from my research with colleagues, particularly Shlomo Silman and Michele Emmer, on auditory deprivation associated with insufficient auditory stimulation, such as that observed in the unaided ear of monaurally fitted individuals with bilateral, symmetric, sensorineural hearing impairment. As will be shown in this text, auditory deprivation may represent one cause of binaural interference. My interest also stems from clinical observations of the many patients with bilateral, symmetric hearing loss who put one or both hearing aids away in a drawer, never to be used again. Undoubtedly, binaural interference furnishes the explanation for some of these cases. Such failure in the use of binaural amplification represents an unjustified expenditure to the individual and a cost to society because of inappropriate and ineffective health care.

We hope the reader will find the existing behavioral and electrophysiological evidence of binaural interference and its impact on auditory function to be compelling. It is our intent that this text on binaural interference will accomplish the following two-fold goal:

1. Provide impetus for pursuing research to enhance (a) understanding of binaural interference in the unaided as well as aided conditions, including its psychoacoustic and physiologic bases; (b) its impact on auditory function; and (c) its management. As with many scientific phenomena, binaural interference is likely to be multifactorial and variable in clinical presentation.
2. Encourage audiologists to explore the possibility of binaural interference when patient complaints suggest this issue, and when performing audiological evaluations. Expanding the screening and diagnostic armamentarium to include procedures to identify and assess binaural interference will lead to the development and implementation of more efficacious management approaches that are targeted to the individual (e.g., eschewing the binaural amplification approach as a one-approach-fits-all with bilateral, symmetric sensorineural hearing loss).

Although we recognize that binaural interference can occur in individuals with cochlear implants, including those with bimodal fittings, the inclusion of binaural interference in individuals with cochlear implants is beyond the scope of this text.

Special appreciation is extended to Lina A.J. Reiss, PhD, who reviewed selected chapters, and to Susan W. Jerger, PhD, for her edits.

It has been a huge honor for me to have the experience of coauthoring a text with Jim Jerger. My heartfelt thanks go to my cherished husband, Shlomo Silman, PhD, for his unwavering and continuous support, guidance, and encouragement over the years, and to my dearly loved brother, Alan K Silverman, MD.

—Carol A. Silverman, PhD, MPH

1

A Brief History of Binaural Interference

VERN O. KNUDSEN

The first published suggestion that there might be such a thing as conflict between the two ears was apparently made in 1939 by Vern O. Knudsen (1893-1974), a world-renowned acoustical physicist at the University of California, Los Angeles. Knudsen is perhaps best known to audiologists as a cofounder of the Acoustical Society of America. Almost 80 years ago, in a paper entitled, "An Ear to the Future," published in the *Journal of the Acoustical Society of America*, Knudsen speculated about the future possibility of binaural hearing aids. He suggested that, although they were the undoubted wave of the future, their value might be limited in some hearing aid users. Knudsen had observed that, in cases of what we now call sensorineural hearing loss, a pitch discrepancy between ears sometimes seemed to generate an *"inter-aural conflict"* if both ears were amplified (Knudsen, 1939). Similar observations were reported in 1949 by Leland Watson and Thomas Tolan (1949). Their warnings were ignored for more than three decades.

In 1971, however, Arkebauer, Mencher, and McCall (1971) reported a curious finding. Previously Harford and Dodds (1966) had measured speech recognition in 29 persons with unilateral hearing loss under two conditions, (1) unaided and (2) aided by a Contralateral Routing of Signal (CROS) input fitted to the poorer ear. This, in effect, created binaural stimulation. In 14 cases, the binaural aided-by-CROS score was better than the unaided score, but in the remaining 15 cases, the unaided score still gave the better result. Reasoning that, in some cases, the impoverished signal provided by the CROS input might have actually interfered with the unaided signal, Arkebauer et al. set out to determine the effect of the input from the poorer ear on the better ear in 10 persons with asymmetric sensorineural loss. They tested speech recognition in the sound field under two conditions: first with the poorer ear open (binaural condition), then with the poorer ear occluded (monaural condition). Speech recognition was assessed with W-22 word lists. Two groups of five individuals each were tested. In both groups, the hearing level on the poorer ear averaged about 60 dB, but in one group, the hearing level on the better ear averaged about 10 dB, whereas in the other group, the average level on the better ear was about 28 dB. The results seemed to confirm the hypothesis of interference from the poorer ear. In eight of the 10 participants, the speech score was better in the occluded (monaural) condition than in the unoccluded (binaural) condition. In the five listeners with only minimal loss in the good ear, the speech score improved by an average of 3.6 % when the poorer ear was occluded. In the five listeners with moderate loss in the better ear, the improvement when the poorer ear was occluded averaged 13.6%. Arkebauer et al. described the effect as, *"detrimental binaural interaction"* (p. 212). Perhaps because of the small number of participants, this study had little impact at the time it was published.

In 1984, the plot began to thicken. Shlomo Silman, Stanley Gelfand, and Carol Silverman reported the results of the analysis of W-22 scores over a 4- to 5-year period for both ears of veterans who had been fitted with a hearing aid monaurally at the Veterans Administration (VA) Hospital in East Orange, New Jersey. Scores did not change very much on the aided ear over the 5-year period, but declined significantly on the unaided ear. The authors termed this "late onset auditory deprivation." Subsequent research confirmed that veterans who had been fitted binaurally initially tended not to show the deprivation effect on either ear. Aside from the obvious implication that binaural fitting should be the fitting method of choice, the deprivation effect emphasized that speech recognition ability is fragile in an ear with unaided sensorineural hearing loss. Could this explain the curious result of the Arkebauer et al. study? Did the greater loss in the poorer-hearing-ear, deprived of stimulation, actually interfere with the speech recognition ability of the better ear in the sound field condition until the poorer ear was plugged? Here was a strong argument for what has come to be called the "auditory deprivation effect" (Silverman & Emmer, 1993) as one possible cause of what we now call "binaural interference."

The term "binaural interference" first appeared in the audiological literature in a 1993 paper by Jerger, Silman, Lew, and Chmiel in the *Journal of the American Academy of Audiology*. This was a series of in-depth case studies of four individuals who showed strong signs of abnormal binaural processing. Data included W-22 scores, the auditory brainstem response (ABR), the auditory middle latency response (AMLR), and a behavioral task involving cued listening to continuous speech discourse in the presence of multitalker babble. The authors concluded that:

> The exact mechanism of the binaural interference effect is not clear. It would appear, however, that by virtue of asymmetric distortion, either on a peripheral or central basis, the input to one auditory pathway suppresses or inhibits the input to the other pathway. (p. 130)

Over the next two decades, research in the area of binaural interference took one of two directions: analysis of either (1) speech recognition scores derived from group studies (Allen, Schwab, Cranford, & Carpenter, 2000; Henken, Waldman, & Kishon-Rabin, 2007; Karsten & Turner, 2000; Leigh-Paffenroth, Roup, & Noe, 2011; McArdle, Killion, Mennite & Chisolm, 2012; Mussoi & Bentler, 2017; Walden & Walden, 2005), or (2) a variety of auditory test data from individual case studies (Bellis, 2002; Carter , Holmes, 2003; Noe, Wilson, 2001; Jerger et al., 1993; Hurley, 1993; Jerger, Silman, Silverman, and Emmer, 2017; Silman, 1995).

GROUP STUDIES

Group studies have generally asked the question, "How many members of the group showed the unexpected pattern of better monaural than binaural scores on a test of speech recognition?" Four of the studies cited above involved testing in the aided condition, whereas the remaining five involved testing in the unaided condition. The percentage of each group showing the binaural interference pattern varied from 0% to 82%, suggesting that many uncontrolled confounding variables were at work among the nine groups. The corrected median prevalence across groups was 19%, which agreed most closely with the experimental results of McArdle et al. (2012). (Table 5–1 in Chapter 5 details these nine studies). Although test conditions varied widely, and prevalence estimates covered a considerable range, two findings were fairly consistent: (1) the observations that the binaural interference pattern was more likely to occur in elderly listeners than in younger adult listeners, and (2) the conclusion that the degree of hearing loss did not appear to be a significant factor influencing prevalence of binaural interference. Finally, McArdle et al. argued persuasively that conclusions regarding the presence of binaural interference derived from aided sound-field testing are questionable unless the non-test ear has been plugged in the monaural test condition in order to prevent the unplugged, non-test ear from artificially inflating the best monaural test score.

Whereas possible binaural interference is an apparently significant issue in hearing aid use (McArdle et al., 2012; Walden & Walden, 2005) it is important to distinguish between binaural interference, in itself, and its possible effect on the hearing aid user. In the latter case, relating to hearing aid use, it is understandable that the "how many" question has been the paramount interest of group studies; but in the former case, relating to binaural interference, in itself, the more important question has been "why" the phenomenon occurs at all. Where in the auditory system does the breakdown appear? Here progress has depended not on group ("how many") studies, but on the analysis of intensive data from individuals who, by careful documentation, have been shown to reflect binaural interference.

CASE REPORTS

The most important difference between group studies and case reports is the extent of documentation of the reality of the binaural interference effect in an individual participant. In group studies, the data are usually confined to the three conventional speech-in-noise scores: monaural right, monaural left, and binaural (or their amplified equivalents, unilateral right, unilateral left, and bilateral). Binaural interference is then defined in an individual participant as the outcome in which the best monaural score exceeds the binaural score.

For the sake of our sanity through all of these numbers, mostly ours but yours as well, when summarizing aided results throughout this book, we will dispense with the distinctions between monaural and unilateral, and between binaural and bilateral. All aided results will still retain the traditional monaural and binaural nomenclature.

However, how can we be sure that this observed difference is not explainable by the error of measurement inherent in the percent correct scores? Here, the Thornton and Raffin (1978) 95% confidence intervals for scores are often consulted. Still one has the uncomfortable feeling that the decision to call an individual result "binaural interference" ought to be based on firmer evidence than two speech-recognition scores.

In case studies, however, the decision to accept test results as indicative of binaural interference is typically based on more than two speech recognition scores. The investigator seeks a common thread across two or more independent measures, and seeks, whenever possible, replicability. Likely suspects are abnormalities in the ipsilateral and contralateral acoustic reflexes, the auditory brain stem response (ABR), the masking level difference (MLD), the auditory middle latency evoked response (AMLR), the auditory late vertex response (ALVR), and directed-report measures of dichotic listening.

An example of a well-documented case study is the report of a 36-year old man with multiple sclerosis by Shlomo Silman (1995). Data are summarized in Figures 1–1A through 1–1E.

During an acute phase of sudden loss of high-frequency hearing sensitivity on the left ear, the average Hearing Level (PTA) fell to 42 dB on the left ear, and the speech recognition score for W-22 words declined to 28% (Figures 1–1A and 1–1B).

In addition, the left contralateral acoustic reflex thresholds (stimulus activation of the left ear) were significantly elevated at all test frequencies and, the reflex decay measures were positive at 500 Hz and 1000 Hz. During a subsequent period of remission (see Figure 1–1B, Retest #1), the high-frequency loss in the left ear improved by 30 to 40 dB at 1000 Hz and above, but did not completely resolve (PTA = 13 dB, W-22 = 82%). The left contralateral acoustic reflex thresholds remained significantly elevated, although the left acoustic-reflex decay results reverted from positive to negative. The ABR was normal on the right ear but absent beyond wave I on the left ear. The ABR to binaural stimulation also showed only wave I (Figure 1–1C). The auditory middle latency response (AMLR) was within normal limits on the right ear, but the Pa component of the MLR was absent from the left ear an (Figure 1–1D).

On a second retest (see Figure 1–1B, Retest #2), the high-frequency component in the left ear had completely resolved, The PTA and W-22 results were still within normal limits on the left ear (PTA = 3 dB; W-22 = 96%), but the amplitude of the Pa component of the AMLR (Figure 1–1E) in both the left ear and binaural conditions was still well below the Pa amplitude on the right ear.

In summary, Figure 1–1B shows that, on the first retest, two independent test results reflected binaural interference, the ABR and the AMLR. On both tests, the monaural result on the right ear was better than on either the left ear or the binaural result. Moreover, the MLR pattern of abnormality was repeated on retest. Note that the conclusion of binaural interference could be made independently of any speech audiometric scores.

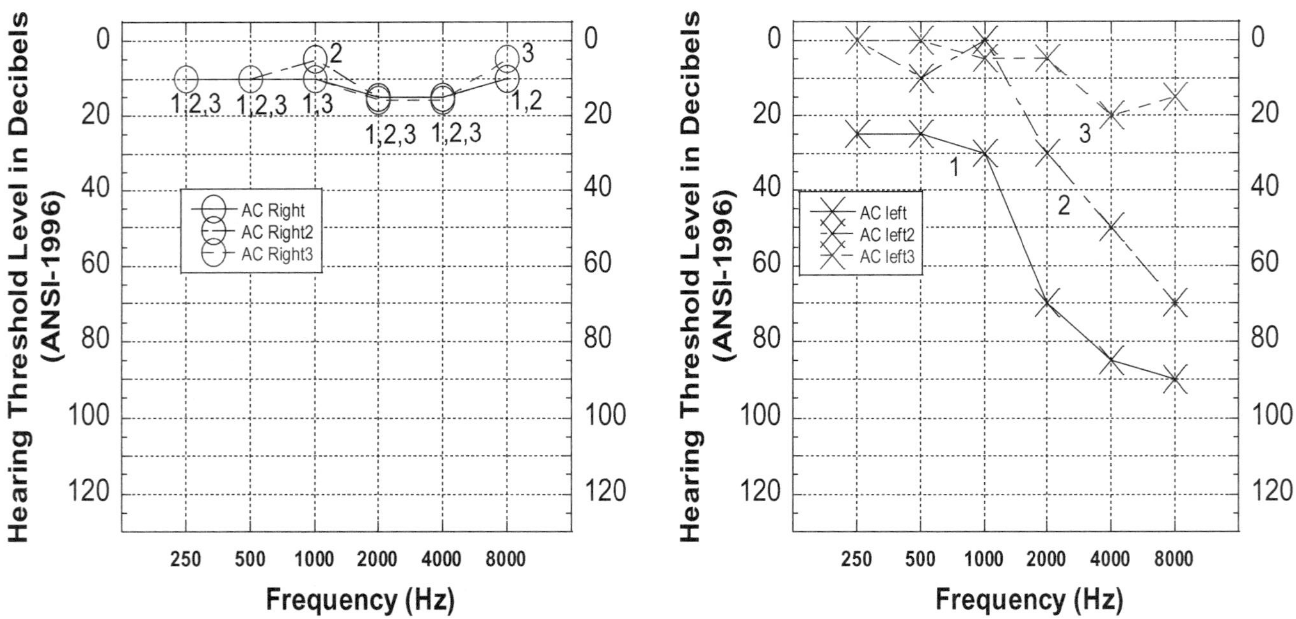

A

Figure 1–1. A. Audiograms of a 36-year-old man with multiple sclerosis. Initial test and two retests. All data in Figure 1–1 have been modified from Silman, S. (1995). Binaural interference in multiple sclerosis: Case study. *Journal of the American Academy of Audiology, 6*, 193–196. *continues*

Initial Test			
Test	**RE**	**LE**	**BIN**
PTA (dB)	12	42	
W-22 (%)	96	28	
First Retest			
PTA (dB)	10	13	
W-22 (%)	96	82	
ABR	WNL	***Wave I Only***	*Wave I Only*
AMLR	Robust Pa	***Absent***	***Absent***
Second Retest			
PTA (dB)	12	3	
W-22 (%)	100	96	
AMLR	Robust Pa	*Weak Pa*	*Weak Pa*

B

Figure 1–1. *continued* **B.** Summary of additional audiometric findings on initial test and two retests. Initial test showed sudden sensitivity loss on left ear and substantial loss on PB score. On retest #1, binaural interference was evident on ABR and MLR evoked responses. On retest #2, the MLR was slightly improved but continued to show a binaural interference pattern. Italics indicate abnormal results. *continues*

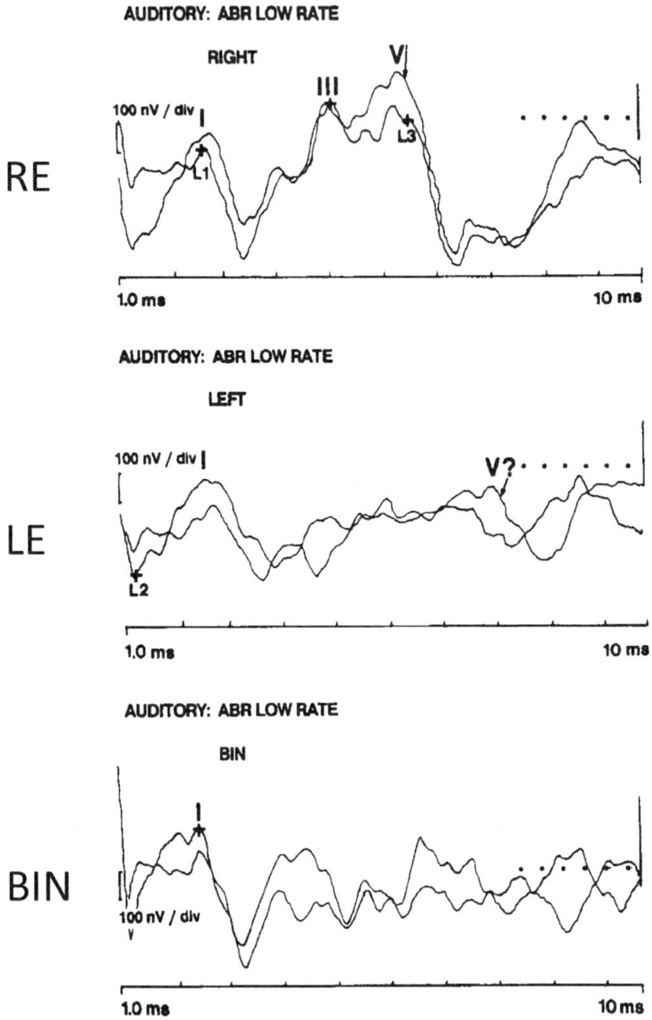

C

Figure 1–1. *continued* **C.** ABR waveforms on retest #1 for RE, LE and BIN stimulation. Waves I, III, and V are present at normal latencies in the right ear, but only wave I is present for left ear and binaural conditions. *continues*

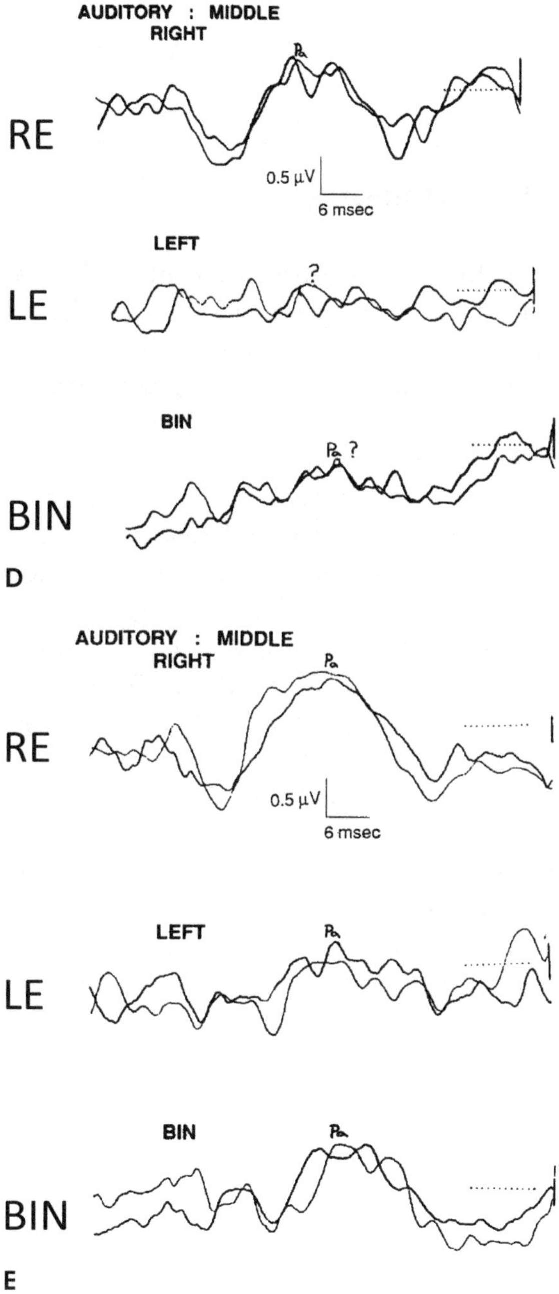

Figure 1–1. *continued* **D.** MLR waveforms on retest #1. Note attenuated Pa peak in BIN condition. Binaural interference is evidenced by the fact that the BIN Pa Peak is not as great as the RE Pa peak. **E.** MLR waveforms on retest #2. There is considerable improvement over result on retest #1, but BIN Pa peak is still substantially less than RE Pa peak.

In Chapter 4, we present a series of such case studies in order to illustrate how the presence of binaural interference may be appropriately documented.

MIRABILE DICTU-KNUDSEN REDUX

We bring this chapter to a close by reporting a recent study that brings us full circle back to Vern Knudsen in 1939. Knudsen's warning that some hearing aid users might not benefit from binaural aids because of an interaural pitch conflict, has recently been verified by Lina Reiss, Jessica Eggleston, Emily Walker, and Yonghee Oh (2016). Their paper is titled "Two Ears Are Not Always Better Than One: Mandatory Vowel Fusion Across Spectrally Mismatched Ears In Hearing–Impaired Listeners." The study compared monaural and binaural vowel classification functions for vowel pair continua in five hearing-impaired listeners. Analysis of their data indicated four trends: (1) similar monaural and binaural functions, (2) ear dominance, (3) binaural averaging, and (4) binaural interference. The latter two findings were observed in three of the five listeners.

Reiss et al. suggest that listeners with hearing impairment may experience abnormal binaural integration of sounds between ears as evident by: (a) abnormally broad fusion of sounds between ears such that sounds of different pitches delivered to the two ears are not perceived as two sounds until the pitch differences are wide, and (b) interaural pitch mismatch, which can result in lack of congruence of spectral information between ears. When the incongruent information is combined in binaural stimulation conditions, the result can lead to a percept that differs from that elicited in the monaural stimulation condition. Indeed, Reiss et al. pose the following questions:

> What are the effects of such abnormal binaural integration on the perception of complex stimuli, such as speech sounds? Can

> abnormal binaural integration account for reduced speech perception benefit, or even interference, with two ears compared to one? (p. 342)

SUMMARY

Almost 80 years ago, when a single hearing aid was still carried in the shirt pocket or in a halter, Vern Knudsen speculated that binaural aids, carried on the head, would someday become the wave of the future. He cautioned, however, that they might not work for all candidates. He had observed a pitch mismatch between the two ears of some hearing aid users, and he thought that might prove to be a problem for successful binaural use.

Since the landmark study of Arkebauer et al. in 1971, there have been a number of studies asking the question, "Are two ears necessarily better than one in all hearing-impaired persons?" The term "binaural interference" first appeared in the audiological literature in the 1993 article by Jerger et al. Since then, research has taken one of two directions: either group studies asking what the prevalence of binaural interference is (the "how many" question), or individual case studies asking what accounts for this apparent failure of the binaural system in some hearing-impaired persons (the "why" question). Events have come full circle with the paper by Reiss, Eggleston, Walker, and Oh (2016), confirming Knudsen's prediction that an interaural pitch conflict may explain at least some cases of binaural interference.

2

Indirect Evidence of Binaural Interference

It is clear from the literature on binaural interference that there is a substantial gap between the theoretical advantage of two hearing aids over one, and the actual preferences of people who buy and use hearing aids. In attempting to clarify this disparity, some investigators have taken one of three indirect approaches: (1) simulation of the effects of asymmetric signal degradation in young adults with normal hearing, (2) retrospective surveys in which a relatively large sample of participants who have already been fitted with two aids are surveyed on what they are actually using in everyday life, (3) field trials in which participants are fitted with either one or two hearing aids, acclimatized to their use, then queried as to which arrangement they prefer.

In the following sections, we summarize recent studies designed to probe binaural interference by taking such indirect approaches.

SIMULATING THE EFFECTS OF ASYMMETRIC SIGNAL DEGRADATION

Anyone who has been involved in a study of individuals drawn from a clinical population is well aware of the difficulties encountered in attempting to control for variables such as age, gender, degree of loss, degree of interaural asymmetry, speech recognition ability on each ear, duration of loss, age of onset of loss, chronological age, cognitive deficit, and other factors specific to the particular problem at issue. This common problem has led some investigators to confront the issue indirectly. One approach has been to simulate the effects of asymmetric signal degradation in young adults with normal hearing.

At Vanderbilt University, Rothpletz, Tharpe, and Grantham (2004) reasoned that binaural interference could be studied more efficiently by simulating the effects of asymmetric signal degradation digitally, and using the degraded signals to test children and young adults with normal hearing. They simulated the effects of sensorineural hearing loss (reduced auditory frequency selectivity, selective threshold elevation, and loudness recruitment) by digitally altering HINT-C sentences presented against 6-talker babble. There were three listening conditions: (a) monaural with mild degradation, (b) binaural with mild degradation in both ears (symmetric degradation), and (c) binaural with mild degradation in one ear and severe degradation in the other ear (asymmetric degradation). All testing was carried out via insert earphones; the problem of excluding the non-test ear in sound field testing did not arise. The authors tested 28 children and 14 young adults, all with normal audiometric findings. Their initial hypothesis, that children would show more bilateral interference from asymmetric signal degradation than adults, was not affirmed by the data, perhaps because the already high signal-to-babble ratio in the children prevented the observation of further decline in performance under the binaural asymmetric degradation condition. In the case of young adults, however, performance was indeed significantly worse in the binaural asymmetrically degraded condition than in the monaural condition. The authors concluded that:

> . . . findings from the current study suggest that asymmetrical signal degradation between the two ears prevents some listeners from capitalizing on the benefit of binaural speech understanding in noise (p. 278).

This conclusion might very well serve as a textbook definition of binaural interference.

It is interesting that, even in the case of young adults with normal audiometric findings, the Rothpletz et al. data were quite variable. Of the 14 young adults (age range from 24 to 29 years) 11 showed poorer binaural than monaural scores, but three showed better binaural than monaural scores. Although the mean binaural interference score was a signal-to-babble ratio of just +1 dB, equivalent to about a 9% decline in speech intelligibility, the

14 individual differences ranged from −2 to +4 dB. If there is so much variability in a homogenous group of young adults, it should not be surprising to find even more variability in elderly persons with hearing loss and variable degrees of cognitive deficit. Rothpletz et al. suggest that a real-life consequence of bilateral interference might make communication difficult when multitasking is involved; for example, while simultaneously listening and taking notes, or following directions.

RETROSPECTIVE SURVEYS

A second approach has addressed the issue indirectly by surveying a large number of persons who are already established hearing aid users. These studies ask the following question directly: "How many people who are actually using amplification prefer one aid instead of two aids?" The surveys may include questions meant to illuminate why the particular choice was made. Table 2–1 summarizes findings from four retrospective studies.

Table 2-1. Preference for One Aid Over Two Aids Across Four Retrospective Surveys

Study	Year	*N*	Preference for One Aid Over Two Aids
Brooks & Bulmer	1981	204	3%
Chung & Stephens	1986	200	19%
Dillon, Birtles, & Lovegrove	1999	4421	20%
Boymans, Goverts, Kramer, Festen, & Dreschler	2009	1000	31%

The number of persons surveyed ranged from 200 to 4,421. Preference for one aid over two aids ranged from 3% to 31%. The advantage of such retrospective studies is that data may be collected on relatively large samples of hearing aid users. The disadvantage is that strict experimental control over data quality is difficult to achieve.

A more controlled version of the retrospective survey was recently carried out in Sweden. Köbler, Lindblad, Olofsson, and Hagerman (2010) brought into the laboratory 22 participants with bilateral, essentially symmetric, hearing loss, who had been initially fitted with binaural amplification: 11 persons maintained their preference for binaural aids whereas 11 persons had developed a preference for just one aid. Participants ranged in age from 33 to 61 years. Experimental measures included binaural masking level differences, speech recognition in noise, dichotic listening tests for both digits and consonant-vowel (CV) syllables, and the SSQ questionnaire [probing speech perception (S), location and spatial orientation (S) and quality of hearing issues (Q)] in the unaided condition. All testing was carried out unaided, via headphones. Whereas the unilateral users generally performed less well on all measures, the difference was particularly striking for the dichotic digits tests. In the free recall condition, for example, the mean score averaged across ears for dichotic digits was 88% for the group preferring bilateral aids, but only 68% for the unilateral preference group. In the directed report condition, comparable scores were 94% for the group preferring binaural aids and 80% for the monaural preference group.

The significantly reduced performance in both the free and directed recall conditions in the monaural preference group, as compared with the binaural preference group, suggests the presence of impaired binaural and central auditory processing in the unilateral group; in contrast, the bilateral preference group performed nearly as well as the normal or near-normal hearing group. The authors postulated that dysfunction of the corpus callosum might be the source of the dichotic deficit. The significantly poorer performance on the speech-in-noise tests in the monaural, as compared to the binaural preference group, also indicated worse central auditory processing in the former than in the latter group.

Noteworthy also was the fact that, although the monaural preference group scored below the binaural preference group on all three categories of the SSQ questionnaire, which queried performance in the unaided condition, the difference was significant only for items in the "Spatial" category, which includes localization, distance, and moving items. On the single item, "locate barking dog," for example, the bilateral group averaged a score of 5.9, whereas the average unilateral group score was only 3.0. The importance of spatial cues in explaining at least some of the basis for monaural versus binaural preference is a recurring theme in this book.

FIELD TRIALS

In a typical field trial, a group of new or recent users is first tested on possible predictor variables, fitted with aids, acclimatized in their use, then recalled and queried on individual preferences. The advantage of this approach is that the experimenter can exercise more precise control over relevant details and procedures, especially the efficacy of potential prediction of which users will ultimately opt for a single aid. The disadvantage is that such studies are typically complicated, time consuming, and expensive to carry out. Table 2–2 summarizes the results of six field trials spanning the years from 1981 to 2011. Preference for one aid over two aids varied from 7% to 61%, a somewhat broader range than the preferences summarized for retrospective studies in Table 2–1.

Certainly, the most comprehensive study in this genre was reported by Cox, Schwartz, Noe, and Alexander (2011). Because many of the previous field-trial preference studies had been con-

Table 2-2. Preference for One Aid Over Two Aids Across Six Field Trials

Study	Year	*N*	Preference for One Aid Over Two Aids
Erdman & Sedge	1981	30	7%
Schreurs & Olsen	1985	30	57%
Day, Browning, & Gatehouse	1988	51	22%
Stephens, Callaghan, Hogan, Rayment, & Davis	1991	29	45%
Vaughan-Jones, Padgham, Christmas, & Irwin	1993	29	61%
Cox, Schwartz, Noe, & Alexander	2011	94	46%

ducted before the advent of modern, technologically advanced aids, Cox et al. reasoned that a new study, using newer aids, might alter findings in favor of greater preference for two aids. They assembled a group of 94 volunteers who agreed to participate in a 12-week field trial. Prefitting questionnaires included items probing lifestyle/demand, as well as positive and negative affect dimensions of personality. Prefitting procedures also included a number of auditory measures thought to be potential predictors of preference for one versus two aids. This test battery included measures of binaural summation, binaural squelch, and dichotic digits testing (free and directed recall conditions). After appropriate fitting of new binaural aids, and orientation to them, the 12-week field trial began. An important feature of this acclimatization period was the use of both structured and unstructured periods of use. During the first three weeks of the total trial period, listening conditions were structured so that use was one week of monaural right, one week of monaural left, and one week of binaural use. In the remaining nine weeks, the listener was free to choose whatever mode of listening was preferred.

Importantly, the comparative cost of one versus two aids was not a factor in the preference. The aids were loaned to the participants for the 12-week trial, and were returned to the experimenters at the conclusion of the trial period. No participant was under any obligation to consider the costs of the aids.

Results failed to meet the investigators' expectation that newer aids would reduce preference for a monaural fitting. One aid was preferred over two aids in 46% of the 94 participants. In general, none of the individual proposed predictor preference variables worked out all that well. The combination of four predictor variables, (unaided scores on the Aversiveness to Sounds subscale, the global Abbreviated Profile of Hearing Aid Benefit (APHAB), binaural summation, and the right ear advantage on the dichotic digits free recall condition) yielded accuracy of preference prediction that was just a bit better (66%) than chance. The details of the findings of this study are quite fascinating and should be consulted in the original publication.

To what extent do the data from these three indirect approaches to binaural interference advance our narrative? The study by Rothpletz et al. (2004) certainly provides fuel for the argument that those persons who understand speech better with one aid than with two are experiencing interference from differential degradation of the quality of the speech signal on one of the two ears. However, to what extent any actual degradation in real life is similar to the digital degradation created by the authors remains an open question.

The retrospective surveys and field trials are generally less helpful because they leave unanswered the degree to which the stated preferences are due to genuine binaural interference versus the many other possible factors that motivate people's choices. Nevertheless, Cox reported that, of the participants who preferred one aid, the following five reasons, from a list of 24 possible reasons, were endorsed by at least 50% of the group. Certainly, item numbers 3 and 4 below are the classical reports of hearing aid users who have been identified as suffering binaural interference.

1. In quiet, I understand speech as well or better when I wear only one hearing aid.
2. My voice sounds more natural / comfortable when I wear only one hearing aid.
3. In noisy situations, I understand speech as well or better when I wear only one hearing aid.
4. One hearing aid helps me as much as two.
5. It's inconvenient to use the telephone when I wear two hearing aids.

We must be content, however, with the conclusion that, in the search for preferences, these indirect approaches leave many questions unanswered.

SUMMARY

This chapter describes three indirect approaches to the question, "Do people who prefer one aid over two aids do so because of binaural interference?" The answer is an unqualified "maybe." The study by Rothpletz et al. showed that, when degrading a binaural speech signal asymmetrically, normal hearing young adults will show what looks very much like binaural interference. However, whether the degradation they created in the laboratory is relevant to what happens in the deprived or otherwise damaged auditory system is debatable.

Both retrospective studies and field trials, over a period of almost 40 years, have shown that, in spite of the undoubted advantages of binaural hearing, an astonishingly high percentage of hearing-impaired persons (median = 45% across the six field trial studies of Table 2–2) prefer one aid among persons who have used or at least sampled the use of two aids. However, here the problem is that there are so many other reasons for such preference that the actual proportional contribution of binaural interference remains unknown.

3

Possible Causes of Binaural Interference

Before commencing this discussion of possible causes of binaural interference, it is useful to review what is known about how the two ears are connected to the two cerebral hemispheres of the brain.

THE WIRING DIAGRAM OF THE AUDITORY SYSTEM

Much of our understanding of how the auditory periphery is functionally linked to the cerebral hemispheres is due to three principal sources: (1) The pioneering studies of patients with temporal lobe tumors by a group of Italian investigators, led by Ettore Bocca (Bocca, Caleraro, Cassinari, & Migliavacca, 1955) (2) the structural model of dichotic listening first proposed by Doreen Kimura of the Montreal Neurological Institute (Kimura, 1961), and (3) the imaging studies carried out by cognitive neuroscientists (Gazzinaga, Ivry, & Mangun, 2002).

Bocca et al. studied speech audiometry in patients with temporal lobe tumors. They showed that, although routine speech audiometric measures were unaffected by the lesions, more difficult speech testing materials proved sensitive to the central disorder. When speech materials were low-pass filtered in order to make them more difficult to understand, scores were poorer on the ear contralateral to the tumor than on the ear ipsilateral to the tumor. This was an early demonstration of the prepotency of the crossed pathways over the uncrossed pathways from the ears to the hemispheres.

Doreen Kimura, working with Brenda Milner at the Montreal Neurological Institute, presented different dichotic digits to both ears simultaneously, that is "dichotically." Her principal interest was the study of patients with temporal lobe epilepsy. However, in the process of standardizing her procedure on young adults without neurological disease, she discovered that the right-ear score tended to be slightly better than the left-ear score. This came to be called the "right-ear advantage" in dichotic listening, although "left-ear disadvantage" would be a better way to put it. In attempting to explain the basis for the right-ear advantage/left-ear disadvantage, Kimura developed and advanced what has come to be called the structural model of dichotic listening. Figure 3–1 illustrates the neural pathways upon which the structural model of dichotic listening is based.

In brief, there are both ipsilateral and contralateral paths from each ear to each hemisphere of the brain. That is, the right ear is connected to the right hemisphere via its ipsilateral path, and to the left hemisphere via its contralateral pathway. Similarly, the left ear is connected to the left hemisphere via its ipsilateral pathway, and to the right hemisphere via its contralateral pathway. The connections from each ear to the hemispheres are largely crossed (70% to 90%), (Lazard, Collette, & Perrot, 2011). Stimulation of either ear alone (monaural condition) will elicit a response in both hemispheres. Yet, if both ears are stimulated simultaneously (binaural condition), the situation becomes immediately much more complex. What is happening in the contralateral pathway suppresses what is happening in the ipsilateral pathway via the corticofugal efferent pathways (Lazard et al., 2011). The right ear input is routed directly to the left hemisphere via its contralateral path, while the left ear input is routed directly to the right hemisphere via its contralateral pathway. Both ipsilateral pathways are suppressed, via efferent (descending) projections from the auditory cortices. Suppression of the ipsilateral ascending pathways by the descending pathways averts a major traffic jam at the cortical level when both ears are stimulated simultaneously. These relations are illustrated in Figure 3–1. Now here is where it begins to get really complicated. Whereas multiple functions of the human organism are represented symmetrically in the brain, speech processing appears to be largely lateralized to the left hemisphere, at least in the 85% to 90% of us who are right handed (Lazard et al., 2011). This may, of course, be an oversimplification; recent research by cognitive neuroscientists, especially imaging studies, has challenged the concept of a strict

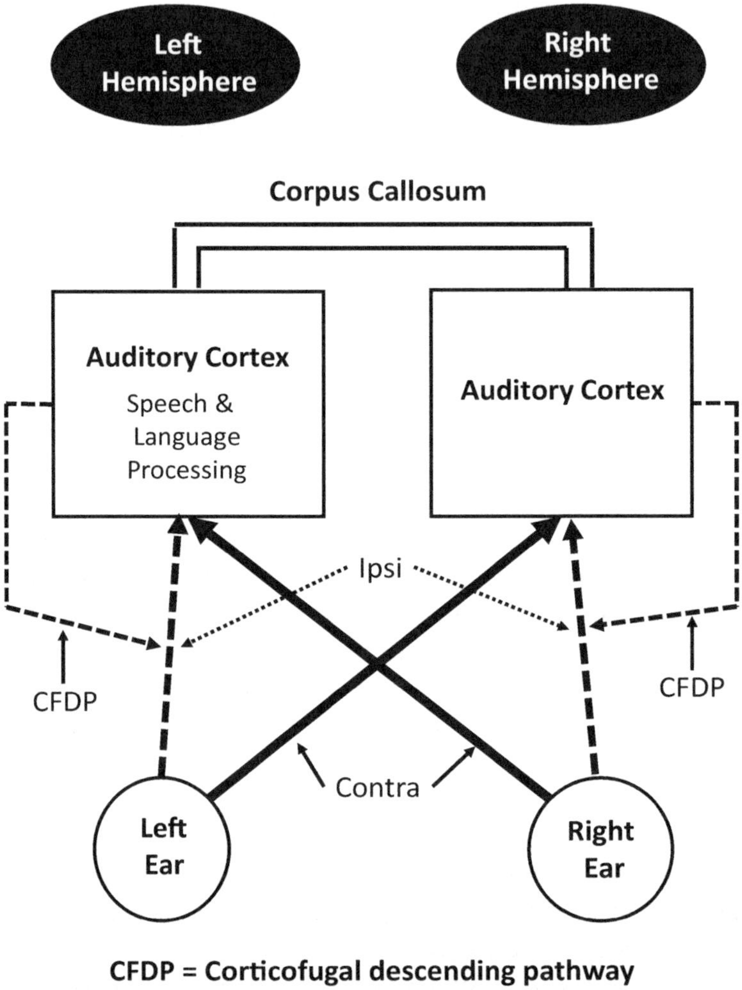

Figure 3–1. Structural model of the auditory pathways from the ears to the hemispheres: how the two ears are connected to the speech processor in the left hemisphere of the brain. There are both crossed and uncrossed routes from each ear to each hemisphere, but the two crossed paths dominate. The uncrossed pathways are inhibited by corticofugal descending pathways. Adapted and modified from p. 169 of Lazard, D., Collette, J., and Perrot, X. (2011). Speech processing: From peripheral to hemispheric asymmetry of the auditory system. *Laryngoscope, 122,* 167–173.

dichotomy of hemispheric specialization of language processing (Gazzinaga, Ivry, & Mangun (2002). Proportional contributions from each hemisphere may be a more realistic description of the process.

In any event, if speech stimuli (e.g., W-22, HINT, QuickSIN) are presented to both ears simultaneously, the input to the right ear travels primarily, but not exclusively, to a speech processing center located primarily in the left hemisphere, whereas the input to the left ear travels primarily, but not exclusively, to the right hemisphere; nevertheless we cannot discount that each hemisphere receives some input from both ears. Although both hemispheres may participate in the processing of the binaural speech input, the structural model assumes that the processing of the two-eared input will be based proportionately on the input from the right ear.

Well, if it all ended that way, there would be no such thing as binaural hearing. Any speech materials presented to both ears simultaneously would only be heard as coming from the right ear. The input to the left ear would be languishing in purgatory in the right hemisphere. However, ever mindful of the need for symmetry in her creation, Mother Nature has provided a way for the full left-ear input to travel from the right hemisphere to the left hemisphere for processing—over a bridge, the corpus callosum. According to the structural model, the left ear input must travel to the right hemisphere first, but then can traverse the corpus callosum to eventually reach the speech-processing center in the left hemisphere. You can see why it is called the structural model. The complexity of the situation may be the price paid for violating the bilateral symmetry of the central nervous system with an overlaid, asymmetric process.

Through the corpus callosal bridge, the left ear input eventually makes its way to the speech/language-processing center in the left hemisphere. However, it takes a little longer for it to make that tortuous journey; not very much (you are not aware of it) but just long enough to lose some information on the way

(Lazard et al., 2011). This slight loss in efficiency of transmission is responsible for the well-known "right-ear advantage" in dichotic listening. The effect is small, but it is always there. The left ear input is always at a slight disadvantage in speech processing.

This right-ear advantage/left-ear disadvantage is revealed by tests of dichotic listening. Here, two different verbal stimuli (e.g., two different words or two different syllables) are presented to the two ears simultaneously. The listener's task is to report back what is heard on each trial. Instructions can either be, (1) "Report back everything you hear." (free report), or (2) "Repeat back only what you hear in the right/left ear." (directed report). Directed report is usually preferred because attention can be better controlled by the test instructions (Bryden, Munhall, & Allard, 1983; J. Jerger, Stach, Johnson, Loiselle, & S. Jerger, 1990). The bottom line here is that the expected result of dichotic testing with verbal targets is a slight right-ear advantage, or more appropriately, a slight left-ear disadvantage. But in some persons, this left-ear disadvantage may be substantial, an abnormal result, indicating that there is a problem with the efficient processing of the left-ear stimulus in the dichotic paradigm, leading perhaps to a substantially delayed and perhaps further degraded input from the left ear to the speech processor in the left hemisphere. Normally this slight left-ear disadvantage is not apparent in the listener's binaural percept. The size of the corpus callosum influences the extent of the left-ear disadvantage. A larger corpus callosum works to offset the left-ear disadvantage by enhancing the velocity of interhemispheric processing of left-ear inputs (Lazard et al., 2011).

Lazard et al. also present two neurophysiologic hypotheses accounting for the left-hemisphere dominance for speech and language processing, and for the routing of left-ear speech input first to the right hemisphere, and then, over the corpus callosum, to the left hemisphere. These hypotheses relate to differing attributes of the auditory cortices in the two hemispheres. One hypothesis emphasizes interhemispheric differences in the temporal domain, such that, in the first stage, speech-language processing in the two hemispheres is symmetric. In the second stage, however, hemispheric processing becomes asymmetric, with the left hemisphere being specialized for short analysis time windows (e.g., for processing of formant and phoneme transitions) and with the right hemisphere being specialized for longer analysis temporal integration time windows (e.g., for processing of the speech envelope, intonation, and prosody).

The second hypothesis emphasizes interhemispheric differences in terms of a trade-off between spectral and temporal resolution, such that the left hemisphere accomplishes better temporal resolution of fast alterations in energy than the right hemisphere; however, the latter accomplishes better spectral resolution than the left hemisphere.

Suppose, however, that something goes wrong in the callosal bridge. Now the input from the left ear is at an even greater disadvantage relative to the input from the right ear. This will produce an even greater left-ear disadvantage. This is sometimes called a "dichotic deficit" because it can be measured by means of a dichotic procedure, such as the Dichotic Digit Test (DDT). All other pertinent variables being equal, (e.g., equal threshold sensitivity in the two ears, for example) dichotic deficits must necessarily appear as left ear disorders in most right-handed persons. However, remember that the problem is in the bridge—the corpus callosum—not in the left ear pathways.

If you were looking for a suspect in the breakdown, known as binaural interference, perhaps you need look no further than a total system in which an asymmetric mechanism has been overlaid on a fundamentally, but not totally, symmetric system (e.g., handedness).

Interestingly, Jacobson, McCandless, and Mahoney (1979) carried out dichotic speech testing in a group of adults with moderate, bilateral, symmetric, sensorineural hearing loss who had been fitted with a hearing aid in the left ear only. Here a left-ear advantage, rather than a right ear advantage was observed on dichotic testing. This finding was in contrast to the expected right-ear advantage observed in: (1) monaurally fitted adults who used the hearing aid in the right ear, (2) participants with normal-hearing sensitivity, and (3) participants with moderate, bilateral, symmetric, sensorineural hearing loss who did not use hearing aids. This unique finding suggests that only fitting the left ear with amplification did, over time, deprive the right ear/left hemisphere of stimulation sufficient to render the left ear/right hemisphere as the dominant side in dichotic testing; a dramatic illustration, perhaps, of the plasticity of the central nervous system. In support of this view, Neuman (2005) has hypothesized that, "changes in auditory system function because of asymmetric auditory stimulation may be differentially affected by greater deprivation of speech signals to the right ear than to the left." (pp. 178-179).

The whole point of this long discussion about the structural model, in conjunction with neurophysiologic explanations, is that it provides audiologists with the ability to roughly estimate where, in this complex structure, the problem of binaural interference seems to be located in a given individual. Our tools for this task are basic pure-tone and speech audiometry, and our site-specific tests: otoacoustic emissions (OAE), the middle ear muscle (MEM) reflexes, the auditory brainstem response (ABR), the auditory middle latency response (AMLR), the late vertex response (LVR) and the various dichotic tests available to us. Another useful measure, cued-listening, is described at length in Chapter 6.

POSSIBLE SOURCES OF BINAURAL INTERFERENCE

Attempts to fully explain why speech recognition can be better monaurally than binaurally in some persons must necessarily await considerably more research. We need more data from the test results of individual cases, bearing on the specific site or sites of disorder underlying the problem. Nevertheless, three prime suspects have already emerged from the literature:

1. Prolonged unilateral deprivation,
2. Age-related changes in interhemispheric transfer via the corpus callosum,
3. Interaural pitch mismatch and binaural fusion due to hearing loss.

Prolonged Unilateral Deprivation

There is substantial literature showing that, if a person with a bilaterally symmetrical hearing loss is fitted with only one hearing aid, the ear deprived of stimulation, that is, the unaided ear, will, over time, show a decline in speech recognition ability that is not accompanied by any decline in pure-tone hearing sensitivity (Silman, Gelfand, & Silverman, 1984). This decrement is observed notwithstanding the occurrence of auditory deprivation many years after the critical period for auditory stimulation. It may be partially or wholly reversible with a change in the hearing aid fitting from monaural to binaural to restore sufficient auditory stimulation to the unaided, formerly deprived, ear (Silverman & Silman, 1990). A factor influencing the magnitude of the deprivation effect is the duration of deprivation (Stubblefield & Nye, 1989). Silman et al. (1984) have suggested that the effect, in all likelihood, represents structural and/or physiological change within the peripheral and/or central auditory system.

In a landmark study of the auditory deprivation effect, Hurley (1993) showed data on nine patients who presented initially with bilaterally symmetrical sensorineural loss and symmetrical speech recognition scores. Each elected to be fitted with a monaural aid, and then, followed yearly, over a period of 4 to 7.5 years, until the speech recognition score on the unaided ear fell significantly below its initial score at the time of the monaural fitting. Each was then fitted with binaural aids and continued to be followed for an additional six months to one year. Although there was some improvement in the speech recognition score on the newly fitted, previously unaided ear, none recovered to the initial score during the short follow-up period. Nevertheless, five of the nine participants elected to continue to use their binaural aids, but the other four rejected them. Three of the four returned the second aid after a 30-day trial. The fourth rejected the second aid after eight months of use. Although we cannot be sure of the actual reasons for rejection of binaural aids in these four cases, binaural interference would certainly be a suspect. The assumption is that the prolonged deprivation of stimulation causes deterioration of the quality of the signal from the deprived ear somewhere in the auditory system. Likely suspects are the cochlea, eighth nerve or low brain stem, although cortical sites may be involved as well.

In a retrospective, longitudinal case study, Boothroyd (1993) followed an individual from age 4 years through age 26 years. The study design parallels an experimental single-subject ABAB design. Initially, the child was monaurally aided in the left ear (phase A in an ABAB design). During that monaural period, phoneme recognition in the unaided right ear declined, reflecting an auditory deprivation effect in that ear. After introduction of binaural amplification (phase B in an ABAB design), phoneme recognition in the formerly unaided right ear improved, reflecting partial recovery. However, the child tolerated binaural amplification for only a brief period, and resumed left monaural amplification (the second phase A in an ABAB design). Phoneme recognition performance in the right ear once again declined, indicating reoccurrence of auditory deprivation. After approximately 14 years of left monaural amplification, the individual suffered an "event" in the left ear that involved deterioration in speech clarity and tinnitus, so she returned to binaural amplification (the second phase B in an ABAB design). Accordingly, phoneme recognition performance in the right ear once again improved over the two-year period of binaural amplification, demonstrating recovery in that ear.

In an interesting pediatric case study, Schoepflin (2007) attempted to establish a more direct link between auditory deprivation and binaural interference. The child, KB, had a severe sensorineural hearing loss, and was fitted monaurally in the right ear at age 1.6 years. Three years later, audiometric testing revealed symmetric hearing loss, but the word-recognition score was substantially poorer in the unaided left ear (40%) than in the aided right ear (88%), suggesting that auditory deprivation had resulted from lack of auditory stimulation in the unaided ear. Binaural amplification was then introduced. Audiometric retesting nine months later revealed essentially no change in hearing sensitivity or word-recognition performance under earphones in either ear. The monaurally aided word-recognition scores mirrored the unaided scores under phones, substantiating the marked word-recognition deficit in the left ear. The binaural, aided word-recognition score of 56% was substantially poorer than the better-ear monaural aided score (90%), indicative of binaural interference. Adverse changes in behavior (e.g., inattentiveness, temper tantrums, and hyperactivity) also followed the introduction of binaural amplification, suggestive of behavioral manifestations of binaural interference.

Evidence that auditory deprivation can lead to changes in the auditory cortex comes from an investigation (Wieselberg & Iório, 2012) of the P300 auditory event-related evoked potential (AERP) in monaurally fitted (mean duration of amplification—about 6 years), binaurally fitted, and never fitted adults with bilateral, symmetric, sensorineural hearing loss. Despite the selection of participants with essentially symmetric word-recognition scores under earphones in quiet, the mean latency of the P300 AERP was significantly longer (5.7 msec longer) in the deprived, unaided ear, than in the fitted ear of the monaurally aided group; no interaural differences in mean latency were observed in the other groups. Also, no interaural differences in mean P300 amplitude were observed in any of the groups. The authors concluded the following:

> The reduction (or increase) in the latency of evoked potentials has been described as a neurophysiologic correlation of neural plasticity and may, often times, precede the behavioral change, which requires longer time to happen, since it may assume the integration of such changes in a perception, besides involving more central cognitive processes (p. 74).

The fact that auditory deprivation can occur from asymmetric auditory input that is unrelated to monaural amplification or from unilateral or asymmetric hearing loss underscores the point that binaural interference can occur independently of amplification. Silman, Jerger, Fanning, Silverman, and Emmer (1998) compared word-recognition performance in the ear habitually used on the telephone with that in the opposite, non-telephone ear. The participants were individuals with adult-onset bilateral, symmetric, sensorineural hearing impairment (suggestive of presbyacusis, or noise-induced hearing loss). The results revealed a significant interaural difference in speech-recognition score; the mean score was 5.1% lower in the non-telephone ear than in the telephone ear. Thus, restriction of telephone use to one ear can yield asymmetric speech-recognition performance that mirrors the asymmetry from monaural hearing-aid use. The asymmetry was more pronounced in the individuals whose pure-tone average (PTA) exceeded 40 dB HL, just as the deprivation effect is more pronounced in individuals with a moderate or worse hearing loss than in those with milder degrees of hearing loss.

Age-Related Changes in Interhemispheric Transfer via the Corpus Callosum

There is converging evidence suggesting that age-related changes affecting interhemispheric transfer via the corpus callosum may underlie some cases of binaural interference. Figure 3–2 lays out the logic of the argument.

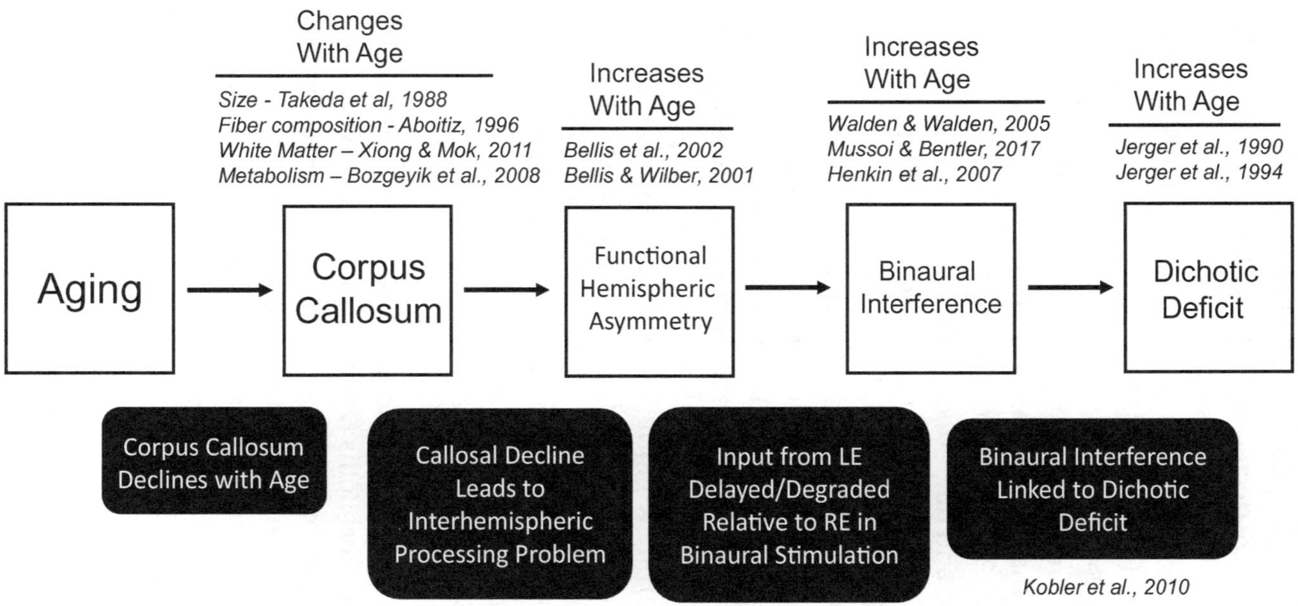

Figure 3–2. Schema suggesting how the effects of aging on the corpus callosum could account for the phenomenon of binaural interference. Age-related changes in the corpus callosum lead to age-related changes in functional hemispheric asymmetry which leads to age-related binaural interference, which is revealed as an age-related dichotic deficit.

As people get older, the corpus callosum functionally declines in four ways: (1) size decreases (Takeda, Yamada, Ono, & Matsuzawa, 1988), (2) fiber composition changes (Aboitiz, Rodriguez, Olivares, & Zaidel, 1996), (3) white matter diminishes (Xiong & Mok, 2011) and, (4) metabolism changes (Bozgeyik, Burakgazi, Sen, & Ogur, 2008). These age-related changes in corpus callosal structure and function lead to an interhemispheric processing problem when the two ears are stimulated simultaneously (Bellis, Nicol, Kraus, 2000; Bellis & Wilber, 2001). The input from the left ear, delayed and degraded by the callosal decline, interferes, rather than supplements, the input from the right ear (Jerger, Alford, Lew, Rivera, & Chmiel, 1995). The result is binaural interference with speech processing, a phenomenon that has also been shown to increase with age (Henkin, Waldman, & Kishon-Rabin, 2007; Mussoi & Bentler, 2017; Walden & Walden, 2005;). It is not surprising, from all of this, that the left-ear disadvantage on dichotic tests, which, by the way, also increases with age (Jerger et al, 1990; Jerger; Darling & Florin,1994), should be linked to binaural interference (Köbler, Lindblad, Olofsson, & Hagerman, 2010).

Perhaps not unrelated to all of this is the frequent observation that, when binaural interference is revealed by speech recognition tests, the best monaural score is usually observed on the right ear (Hill & Purdy, 2011; Jerger, Silman, Lew, & Chmiel, 1993; Walden & Walden, 2005;).

Possibly no one has provided a better description of binaural interference than Teri Bellis (2002). In her book, "When the Brain Can't Hear," she reports on "Ralph," an elderly, reluctant hearing aid user. He was provided with binaural aids for trial but found them impossible to use in noisy situations. On the verge of giving up on hearing aids entirely, and returning both aids to the dispenser, he decided to try wearing just one aid. The right ear seemed to work best. Dr. Bellis reported the following:

> To his extreme surprise, not only was wearing the right aid tolerable, he actually liked it. With a proud grin, he reported how

> he experienced a significant improvement in his listening and understanding abilities when using the hearing aid in just his right ear. (p.158)

All of which leads to the question, "Does decline of callosal efficiency with age account for binaural interference in some elderly persons?"

This explanation fails, of course, to account for the occasional finding of binaural interference in younger individuals. In these cases, there is often a history of cerebrovascular insult to the brain, or other neurological disease, or subtle congenital malformations in callosal efficiency.

Interaural Pitch Mismatch and Binaural Fusion Due to Hearing Loss

The study by Reiss, Eggleston, Walker, and Oh (2016) described toward the end of Chapter 1, and elaborated here, suggests that, binaural interference, in some listeners with hearing impairment, may be explained by abnormally broad binaural fusion of sounds between ears, such that sounds that are disparate, rather than similar, in pitch are perceived as a single sound. Reiss, Eggleston, Walker, and Oh (2016) compared monaural and binaural vowel classification functions for vowel pair continua in five older adult listeners (68 to 80 years of age) with bilateral, essentially symmetric, moderately severe hearing impairment, who were users of binaural hearing aids. As vowel recognition is essentially based on perception of the first and second formant frequencies (F1 and F2), each synthetic vowel was presented with F1 at a frequency that varied between the F1 for one member of the continuum vowel pair (e.g., /ɪ/) to the F1 for the other member of the vowel continuum pair. The five sets of synthetic vowel pairs had essentially similar F2 values for the two vowels within the set but different F1 values (F3 and F4 were held constant). The transition in F1 occurred in small frequency steps between that for one member of a synthetic vowel pair (e.g., /ɪ/) and that for the other member of a vowel continuum pair. The listener was furnished with exemplar words for each vowel continuum pair (e.g., "hid" and "heed" for the /ɪ/ and /i/ synthetic vowels). For each synthetic vowel presented, the listener was instructed to identify the synthetic vowel by choosing one of the members of a given exemplar pair (a two-alternative, forced-choice task). The synthetic vowels were presented in sound field in the right and left monaurally aided conditions and in the binaurally aided condition. During the monaurally aided condition, the contralateral ear was plugged and muffed. Graphs were constructed (vowel classification functions) showing the percentage of time a synthetic vowel was identified to be one of the vowel continuum pair (e.g., /i/ as in "heed"), for each F1 step, for each of the three aided conditions. The steepness of the function indicated the discrimination ability, with steep functions indicating good performance and consistency in discrimination between the two vowel pairs, and shallow functions indicating difficulty in discrimination, that is, all the stimuli sounded similar.

Reiss et al. (2016) concluded that some of the vowel classification patterns reflected binaural interference, especially when there was asymmetry between ears, and one ear had better discrimination and steeper functions than the other ear. Analysis of their data for the users of binaural hearing aids indicated four trends in binaural spectral integration of speech input from the two ears: (1) similar monaural and binaural functions; (2) ear dominance, whereby the binaural pattern is very similar to one of the monaural patterns, (3) binaural averaging, whereby the binaural pattern falls in between the two monaural patterns; and (4) binaural interference in which the binaural pattern differs significantly from both monaural patterns, and also demonstrates poorer speech-discrimination performance than either monaural pattern. Reiss et al. suggest that the averaging pattern may also reflect a form of binaural interference because discrimination performance in the binaural condition is intermediate between those for the two monaural patterns, suggesting poorer speech discrimination ability in the binaural condition than in the best monaural condition. Averaging and interference patterns each were observed in three of the five listeners; two of the three displayed averaging and/or interference patterns for at least two vowel pairs. The findings of this study not only document binaural interference at the level of one phoneme/frequency region, but also show that an interference pattern seen at one phoneme/frequency region in a listener may not be seen at other phoneme/frequency regions. Indeed, interference at one phoneme/frequency region can occur with a binaural pattern that is similar to the two monaural patterns at other phoneme/frequency regions. In Chapter 6, we describe the relation between these binaural interference patterns on the vowel classification functions and abnormally broad binaural fusion.

Here, the most likely suspects are the cochlea, the eighth nerve, or, more likely, the mechanism in the low brain stem that compares and integrates the inputs from the two auditory nerves.

SUMMARY

The basic auditory system is symmetric. Each ear connects to each cerebral hemisphere via both an ipsilateral and a contralateral pathway, but it is clear that the contralateral pathway to each hemisphere is dominant. The processing of speech by the brain is, however, asymmetric. In right-handed persons, most of the processing of speech is carried out by structures located in the auditory cortex in the left hemisphere. Because of the prepotency of the contralateral over the ipsilateral pathways from ear to hemisphere, the right ear input enjoys a slight advantage over the left-ear input in the processing of speech input. In order to reach the speech-processing center in the left hemisphere, the left ear input must travel, first to the right hemisphere, then cross over to the left hemisphere via a bridge, the corpus callosum. This gives rise to a slight right-ear advantage/left-ear disadvantage, a phenomenon demonstrable in dichotic listening tests. The effect is small, almost negligible, in young adults, but increases in some elderly persons, probably as a result of age-related changes in the corpus callosum. These factors may be complicit in the various manifestations of binaural interference.

There are three likely candidates to explain the basis for binaural interference in elderly persons: (1) prolonged unilateral deprivation; (2) age-related changes in interhemispheric transfer of speech stimuli via the corpus callosum; and (3) interaural pitch mismatch due to hearing loss.

All three will profit from further research, but there is ample evidence that each must be seriously considered. All three may be responsible for variations in the expression of the phenomenon.

4

Illustrative Cases

In the following sections, we present data from a series of four cases illustrating audiological findings in persons with clear evidence of binaural interference. They cover the age range from 66 to 90 years. For assistance with the many abbreviations in the figures, please consult Table 4–1.

Please note as you review these cases, that none would have been identified by what has regrettably become the standard audiological assessment in too many clinics, namely, air, bone, and PB scores for right and left ears. At the very least, there should be a binaural test employing the same words or sentences used to evaluate each ear separately.

We grant at the outset that the busy clinician is likely to have neither the time nor the necessary equipment to carry out

Table 4–1. List of Abbreviations Used in Summarizing Results of Audiometric Testing

ABN	Abnormal
ABR	Auditory Brain Stem Response
AERP	Auditory Event-Related Potential
ABS	Absent
ALVR	Auditory Late Vertex Response
AMLR	Auditory Middle Latency Response
dB	Decibel
ID	Identification
LE	Left Ear
MCR	Message-to-Competition Ratio
PB	Phonemically Balanced
PTA	Pure-Tone Average (Mean HL in dB across 500, 1000, and 2000 Hz)
RE	Right Ear
SSI	Synthetic Sentence Identification
WNL	Within Normal Limits

the fairly thorough testing regimens described for some of these cases. The important point is to understand the concept of binaural interference, appreciate how it can be evaluated in a research setting, understand how it is likely to impact the life of patients, and learn best approaches to treatment. See more on these issues in Chapter 7.

CASE REPORTS

Ordinarily, we expect that the left ear input will be the culprit in cases of binaural interference. But, in the first two cases presented here, there were unique problems with right-ear input which, in effect, reversed that expectation.

Case #1: Elderly—Gradual Onset of Hearing Loss

A 71-year-old woman reported a bilateral hearing problem, growing gradually worse over the past 15 years. Ten years earlier, she had been fitted with a hearing aid on the left ear and had worn it successfully since then. She now complains that the aid is no longer as useful as it was earlier. In view of this history, it is possible that the right ear usefulness declined over the 10-year period of monaural use due to the deprivation effect described in Chapter 3. This would explain the present finding that the left ear proved to yield a stronger monaural aided response than the right ear. As noted earlier in Chapter 3, the right ear is usually the better ear when binaural interference is observed.

Figures 4–1A and 4–1B summarize the relevant audiological data. The audiograms show a bilateral, moderately severe, symmetric sensorineural loss, sloping gradually from low to high frequencies. Pure-tone averages (PTA), based on the average of losses at 500, 1000, and 2000 Hz are 65 dB HL on the right ear and 67 dB HL on the left ear. The speech recognition scores for

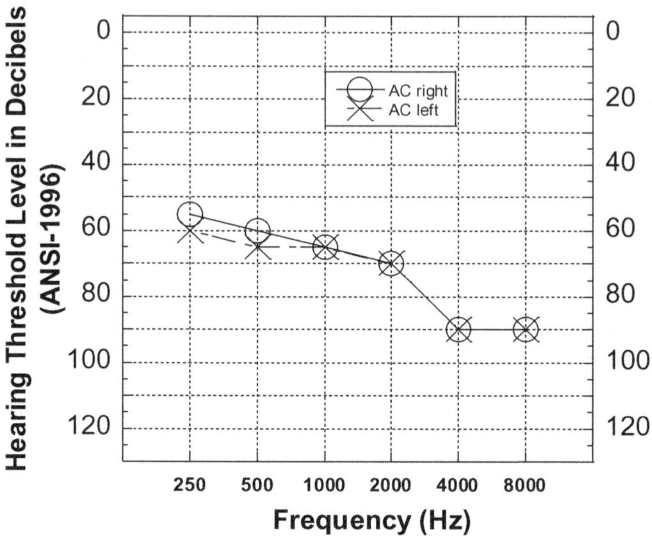

Figure 4–1A. Audiograms of right and left ears of Case #1. Modified from Jerger, J., Silman, S., Lew, H., and Chmiel, R. (1993). Case studies in binaural interference: Converging evidence from behavioral and electrophysiological measures. Journal of the *American Academy of Audiology, 4,* 122–131.

W-22 words in quiet are markedly asymmetric: 0% for the RE and 48% for the LE. The two ears were fitted with binaural aids, and the three conditions, aided right, aided left, and aided binaurally were tested in the sound field. The loudspeaker delivering the W-22 words was oriented facing the listener at 0° azimuth. Results showed that the left monaural score increased by 18% to 66%, the right monaural score remained at 0%, and the aided binaural score was 20%. The reliability of this binaural score was assessed by repeating the binaural-aided condition after a rest period of one hour. This second score was unchanged at 20%.

Please note that the aided left-ear score was 46% better than the binaural score. If the monaural right ear score were having no

Procedure	RE	LE	BIN
PTA (dB)	65	67	
PB Words in Quiet (%)	0	48	
Aided Words in Quiet (%)	0	66	20

Figure 4–1B. Summary of additional audiometric findings in Case #1. Binaural Interference is indicated by the fact that the BIN PB score (20%) is 46% worse that the LE PB score (66%). Modified with permission from Jerger, J., Silman, S., Lew, H., and Chmiel, R. (1993). Case studies in binaural interference: Converging evidence from behavioral and electrophysiological measures. *Journal of the American Academy of Audiology, 4*, 122–131.

effect on the binaural aided score, then the binaural score should have been as good as—rather than markedly worse—than the left monaural aided score. However, it was actually much worse than the monaural left score, less by 46%. It is not unreasonable to suppose that adding input from the poorly performing right-aided ear adversely impacted performance in the binaural aided condition. This is the basic nature of binaural interference.

For what it is worth, the 46% difference between the best monaural score, (66%) and the binaural score, (20%) was statistically significant, falling outside the Thornton and Raffin (1978) 95% confidence interval. Nevertheless, in succeeding pages we hope to convince you that a comprehensive auditory test battery is a better way to verify the reality of true binaural interference than comparison of speech-recognition scores based on 95% confidence intervals.

This case illustrates the bare minimum amount of information necessary to detect the possibility of binaural interference. It tells us little, however, beyond the fact that binaural interference has been detected. We urge the reader not to view binaural interference as a phenomenon affecting speech recognition only in the aided condition. In the case study presented in the editorial, in the Journal of the American Academy of Audiology by Jerger, Silman, Silverman, and Emmer (2017), binaural interference was demonstrated in a young adult on speech-recognition testing in noise under headphones, by the binaural score of 78% that was 14% poorer than the better monaural score (right ear). In subsequent case studies in this chapter, we show how gathering additional site-specific information beyond traditional speech-recognition assessment can tell us more about where the problem lies within the auditory system.

Case #2: Elderly—Left-Sided Cerebrovascular Insult

This 80-year-old man had suffered an earlier left-sided cerebrovascular insult. This naturally had an adverse effect on speech materials presented to the right ear. Ordinarily, in cases of binaural interference, it is the left ear that is most likely to be affected. In this patient, however, the cerebrovascular accident (CVA) on the left hemisphere no doubt adversely affected the input from the right ear substantially, leaving the left as the better ear. Again, as in Case #1, this unique circumstance yielded a result counter to the usual expectation that the right ear will be the better ear when binaural interference is detected.

Figures 4–2A and 4–2B summarize the audiological findings. The audiograms show steeply sloping loss patterns, with somewhat greater low frequency hearing loss on the right than the left ear. The PTAs are consistent with a moderate hearing loss,

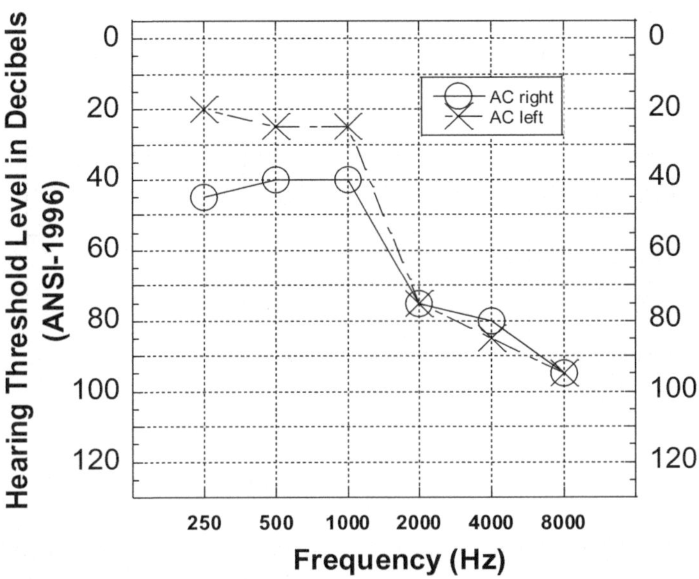

Figure 4–2A. Audiograms of right and left ears of Case #2. Modified from Jerger, J., Silman, S., Lew, H., and Chmiel, R. (1993). Case studies in binaural interference: Converging evidence from behavioral and electrophysiological measures. *Journal of the American Academy of Audiology, 4,* 122–131.

bordering on moderately severe on the right ear. The W-22 scores in quiet are worse on the right than on the left ear. The interaural difference is 44%. Binaural aids were fitted and W-22 scores were obtained again for the three standard conditions. The left monaural aided score (76%) was similar to that in the unaided condition (80%); the score for the right ear declined significantly from 36% in the unaided condition to 8% in the monaural aided condition. In the aided binaural condition, the W-22 score (54%) was significantly lower than the best (left) monaural aided score (76%). A retest of the binaural condition one hour later gave an even poorer binaural score (38%). It is interesting to note that

Procedure	RE	LE	BIN
PTA (dB)	52	42	
PB Words in Quiet (%)	36	80	
Aided PB words in Quiet (%)	8	76	54

Figure 4-2B. Summary of additional audiometric findings in Case #2.

although the right ear showed essentially no aided word recognition, the presence of its input in the binaural condition lowered what should have been a simple repeat of the better (left ear) monaural aided condition from 76% to 54%. Thus, the mere presence of the almost unintelligible right ear input in some way interfered with the processing of the left-ear input in the binaural condition. This is reminiscent of the earlier observations of Arkebauer, Mencher, and McCall, (1971).

In search of an electrophysiological correlate of binaural interference in this patient, we next studied auditory middle latency (AMLR) evoked responses from 19 active scalp electrodes in the three standard conditions: monaural right, monaural left, and binaural signal presentation. Stimuli were brief 1000 Hz tone pips. Pip duration was 5 msec; 1000 consecutive pips were averaged. This procedure normally yields an evoked waveform showing a positive peak (Pa) at a post-stimulus latency of about 35 msec. As with speech recognition, marked interaural asymmetry was observed for Pa peak amplitudes. We found Pa peak amplitudes to be 1.83 μV for left ear stimulation, 0.90 μV for right ear stimulation, and 0.97 μV for binaural stimulation. The presence of the right ear stimulation lowered the binaural peak amplitude in the binaural condition almost 50%, (reduction of 0.86 μV) compared to the 1.83 μV peak in the left ear condition. The actual AMLR waveforms are shown in Figure 4–2C. The fact that the Pa peak of the AMLR was robust for left ear stimulation but substantially attenuated for right ear stimulation is consistent with a problem at the level of the primary auditory cortex on the left

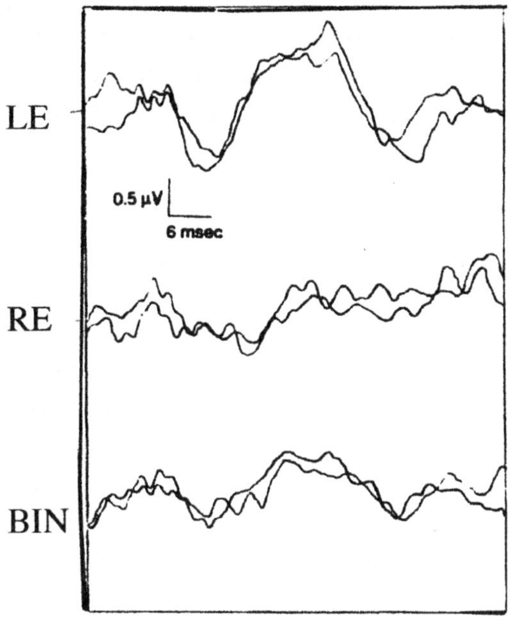

Figure 4–2C. AMLR Waveforms for Case #2. Compare LE amplitude with BIN amplitude. Binaural interference is evident in the AMLR peak Pa amplitudes. The voltage at the BIN peak is only 50% of the voltage at the LE Pa peak. Modified from Jerger, J., Silman, S., Lew, H., and Chmiel, R. (1993). Case studies in binaural interference: Converging evidence from behavioral and electrophysiological measures. *Journal of the American Academy of Audiology, 4,* 122–131.

hemisphere because the MLR response from left ear/right hemisphere stimulation was robust. These audiological findings are consistent with the history of left CVA. They are also consistent with binaural interference in which the right ear input interferes with the left ear input. In this 80-year-old man we have, then, evidence of binaural interference from both behavioral and electrophysiological measures. The W-22 score declined from 76%, when only the left ear was aided, to 54/38% when both ears were aided. Similarly, the amplitude of the AMLR declined from 1.83 μV, when only the left ear was stimulated, to 0.97 μV, when both ears were stimulated.

Case #3: Elderly—Gradual Onset of Mild Hearing Loss

This 81-year-old man reported a gradual onset of mild hearing difficulty for 10 years. Difficulties have been noted only in certain social situations. He had never worn hearing aids but thought that he might be ready. Figure 4–3A shows the pure-tone audiograms. The right ear shows a typical presbyacusic pattern, sloping downward from borderline normal-hearing threshold levels in the low frequency range to essentially moderately severe loss in the high-frequency region. The loss is slightly greater on the left ear above 1000 Hz. Figure 4–3B summarizes the remaining audiological findings. Speech recognition scores for PB words in quiet were 100% on the right ear but only 60% on the left ear, in keeping with the greater high frequency loss on the left side. The auditory brain stem response (ABR) was within normal limits on the right ear, the left ear, and binaurally. The actual ABR waveforms for the three conditions are shown in Figure 4–3C. Note that the wave V amplitude is substantially greater in the binaural condition than in either monaural condition. The AMLR, however, showed the first sign of an interference issue. Figure 4–3D shows the actual AMLR waveforms. For the right ear, the waveform showed a

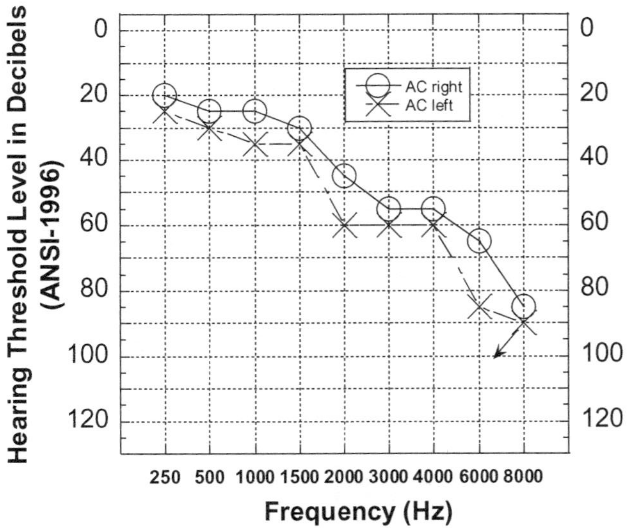

Figure 4–3A. Audiograms of right and left ears of Case #3. Modified from Jerger, J., Silman, S., Lew, H., and Chmiel, R. (1993). Case studies in binaural interference: Converging evidence from behavioral and electrophysiological measures. *Journal of the American Academy of Audiology, 4*, 122–131.

Procedure	RE	LE	BIN
PTA (dB)	32	42	
PB Words in Quiet (%)	100	60	
ABR (microvolts)	WNL	WNL	WNL
AMLR (microvolts)	1.6	0	0

Figure 4–3B. Summary of additional audiometric findings in Case #3. ABR waveforms were all within normal limits (WNL), AMLR Peak PA amplitude was 1.6 μV for RE stimulation, but there was no Pa peak in either the LE or BIN waveforms. Modified from Jerger, J., Silman, S., Lew, H., and Chmiel, R. (1993) Case studies in binaural interference: Converging evidence from behavioral and electrophysiological measures. *Journal of the American Academy of Audiology, 4*, 122–131.

well-formed Pa component, with a peak amplitude of 1.6 μV. But tone pips to the left ear, and pips to both ears (binaural presentation), showed no MLR response. Strong evidence for binaural interference lies in the fact that, even if the left ear were incapable of an AMLR response because of the greater high frequency sensitivity loss, the binaural result should have been a repeat of the right ear result. The lack of any response in the binaural condition can best be explained as a binaural interference effect of left ear

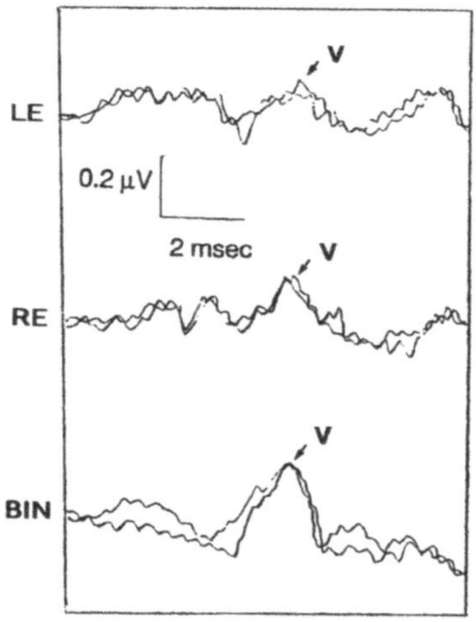

Figure 4–3C. ABR waveforms for Case #3. Note that peak-to-peak wave V amplitude of BIN waveform is larger than in either RE or LE ABR waveforms. Modified from Jerger, J., Silman, S., Lew, H., and Chmiel, R. (1993). Case studies in binaural interference: Converging evidence from behavioral and electrophysiological measures. *Journal of the American Academy of Audiology, 4,* 122–131.

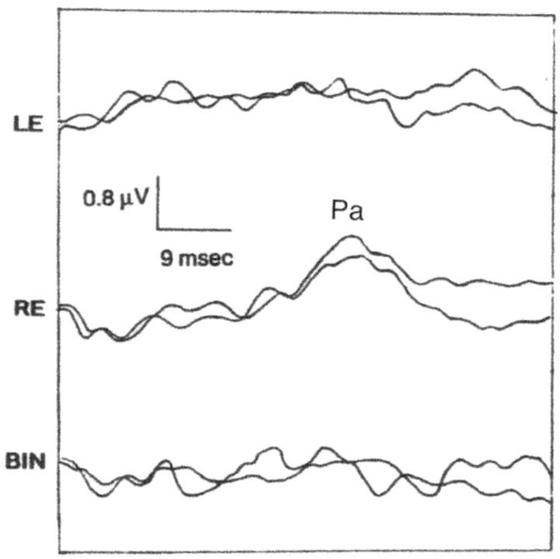

Figure 4–3D. AMLR waveforms of Case # 3. Note well-formed Pa peak on RE waveform, but total lack of Pa peak in either LE or BIN conditions. Modified from Jerger, J., Silman, S., Lew, H., and Chmiel, R. (1993). Case studies in binaural interference: Converging evidence from behavioral and electrophysiological measures. *Journal of the American Academy of Audiology, 4,* 122–131.

processing on the AMLR. The combination of normal ABRs and abnormal MLRs suggests an interference problem at the level of the auditory cortex, the site posited in Case #2.

Case #4: Elderly—Gradual Onset of Hearing Loss Following Aspirin Therapy

This 90-year old woman had a 13-year history of gradual loss of hearing in both ears following aspirin therapy for shoulder pain. At age 87, she had been fitted with binaural aids. She now complained that the aids were unsatisfactory, especially in the presence of background noise. There was no history or obvious evidence of stroke, dementia, neurologic or other systemic disease. Her history was otherwise negative save for hormone therapy for osteoporosis. She was active and in good general health. Figure 4–4A shows her audiograms. The pure-tone levels on both ears revealed a moderate bilaterally symmetrical loss, sloping upward from 250 to 2000 Hz, then sloping sharply downward from 2000 to 8000 Hz. Figure 4–4B summarizes additional audiometric findings. The PTAs were essentially symmetric.

As with the other cases, PB recognition scores in quiet showed significant interaural asymmetry; the score was significantly worse in the left than the right ear. Both scores were remarkably good for a ninety-year-old person, but the score for the left ear was definitely down somewhat relative to that for the right ear. Aided Synthetic Sentence Identification (SSI) scores in the presence of single-talker competition in the sound field reflected possible binaural interference; the right aided score was 80%, the left aided score was 20%, and the binaural aided score was 50%. Otoacoustic emissions, ABR, AMLR, and the auditory late vertex response (ALVR) (Figure 4–4C) were all within normal limits on both ears. Nevertheless, aided Synthetic Sentence Identification (SSI) scores in the presence of single-talker competition in the sound field reflected possible binaural interference;

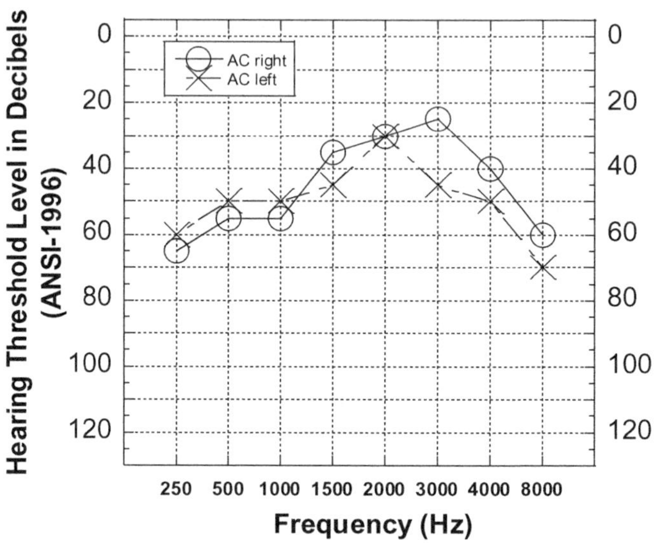

Figure 4-4A. Audiograms of right and left ears of Case #4. Modified with permission from Chmiel, R., Jerger, J., Murphy, E., Pirozzolo, F., and Tooley-Young, C. (1997). Unsuccessful use of binaural amplification by an elderly person. *Journal of the American Academy of Audiology, 8,* 1–10.

the right aided score was 80%, the left aided score was 20%, and the binaural aided score was 50%.

If you run scores like this past a psychologist, chances are you will hear a lot about how such findings can be explained by age-related cognitive changes in attention and memory. They are usually right, but there are exceptions. The patient in Case #4 is one of them. To evaluate the possibility that the apparent binaural interference could be explained by a cognitive variable, we set out to test dichotic listening for SSI sentences as we manipulated the memory and attentional demands on the listener.

As a necessary first step, we determined that our nonagenarian listener was able to identify all sentence when they were presented monaurally, both when they were presented

Procedure	RE	LE	BIN
PTA (dB)	47	43	
PB Words in Quiet (%)	96	76	
Aided SSI Sentences In Competition (%)	80	20	50

Figure 4–4B. Summary of additional audiometric measures for Case #4. Modified from Chmiel, R., Jerger, J., Murphy, E., Pirozzolo, F., and Tooley-Young, C. (1997). Unsuccessful use of binaural amplification by an elderly person. *Journal of the American Academy of Audiology, 8*, 1–10.

Procedure	RE	LE
Otoacoustic Emissions	WNL	WNL
ABR	WNL	WNL
AMLR	WNL	WNL
ALVR	WNL	WNL

Figure 4–4C. OAEs, ABRs, AMLRs, and ALVRs were all within normal limits. Modified from Chmiel, R., Jerger, J., Murphy, E., Pirozzolo, F., and Tooley-Young, C. (1997). Unsuccessful use of binaural amplification by an elderly person. *Journal of the American Academy of Audiology, 8*, 1–10.

singly and in pairs. First, we presented one sentence at a time to each ear separately. Identification scores were 100% in both ears. Then we presented two sentences in succession on each trial. This task placed a greater demand on short-term memory, and scores fell to 90% on the right ear and 80% on the left ear; still reasonably good performance on both ears for a 90-year-old woman. Figure 4–4D summarizes results of four separate dichotic tests. First, we presented the sentences dichotically, in the free-report mode. Here, scores were 90% for the right ear, but only 10% for the left ear, an interaural difference of 80%. This suggested a significantly abnormal left-ear disadvantage. The next step was to repeat the same dichotic procedure, with the same sentences, in a different random order, but employing the directed-report mode. We reasoned that, if the previous result (RE=90%, LE=10%) were contaminated by an attentional deficit, the effect of changing to the directed attention mode should improve the left-ear score. However, that did not happen. The

Procedure	RE	LE
Dichotic Sentence ID-Free Report (%)	90	10
Dichotic Sentence ID-Directed Report (%)	90	10
Dichotic Sentence ID Pre-Cued	100	10
Dichotic Sentence ID Post-Cued	100	10

Figure 4–4D. Dichotic measures for SSI Sentence identification showed a severe left-ear disadvantage for verbal materials. Modified from Chmiel, R., Jerger, J., Murphy, E., Pirozzolo, F., and Tooley-Young, C. (1997). Unsuccessful use of binaural amplification by an elderly person. *Journal of the American Academy of Audiology, 8*, 1–10.

interaural difference remained at 80%. Perhaps, we thought, there might be a severe memory problem in the directed-report mode, such that, during the testing, she lost track of which ear she had been directed to attend. We thought we might help her in the memory department by precuing the ear-to-be attended before each trial. Again, however the left ear score remained at 10%. All right, we said, we will randomly alter the ear to be attended, but will postcue that information after each trial of word pairs has been presented. This task requires that the listener must first process both sentences of the dichotic presentation. After being postcued, the listener must then retrieve the two-dichotic sentences while recalling to memory which ear was designated by the postcued instruction. She must then make the appropriate response. This, we reasoned, should put such a strain on her declining cognitive resources that her performance would surely crash in both ears. However, the same 90% to 10% scores were obtained. We concluded that the substantial dichotic interaural difference could not be easily explained by declines in either memory or attention.

Perhaps, however, it could be explained by age-related decline in corpus callosal function. To investigate this possibility, we gathered P300 auditory event-related evoked potential data from each ear. In the P300 paradigm, a series of auditory events is presented to the listener. Some of the events are designated as targets, the remainder as nontargets. The listener's task is to press a response button each time a target event is heard. While this is going on, the brain electrical activity evoked by each event is recorded from scalp electrodes affixed to the skull. These individually evoked electrical voltages, recorded after each trial, are averaged separately for targets and nontargets. If the a priori probability of a target event is low (10% to 30% of the entire series), the average evoked response to the target events will show a positive peak at a post-stimulus onset latency varying from 300 to 900 milliseconds, depending on the nature of the auditory events and the difficulty of the task (Picton, 2011).

Within the context of the P300 paradigm, we constructed a dichotic PB word (CVC) design. Pairs of PB words were presented on each trial. A complete test condition consisted of 300 trials. On each trial, the listener heard a PB word in one ear and a different PB word in the other ear. There were two separate conditions, verbal targets and non-verbal targets. The aim here was to evaluate the integrity of both the right-ear-to-left-hemisphere pathway and the left-ear-to-right hemisphere pathway. As noted in Chapter 3, current thinking emphasizes interhemispheric differences in terms of a trade-off between spectral and temporal resolution, the left hemisphere is better at temporal resolution of fast alterations in energy (e.g. a word), and worse at spectral resolution, whereas the right hemisphere is better at spectral resolution (e.g., voice gender), but worse at temporal resolution. To test the right-ear-to-left-hemisphere system, we employed a task requiring a decision on each trial in which target words were words that rhymed with "book," an essentially phonological analysis. In order to test the left-ear-to-right-hemisphere system, we presented the same words again, but the task was to decide whether the talker was a male or a female, essentially a spectral analysis of voicing. In both conditions, nontargets were simply randomly chosen PB words with no additional significance. For the verbal condition, all words, target and nontarget, were spoken by a male talker. In the nonverbal condition, nontarget words were spoken by the same male talker, but targets were randomly chosen PB words spoken by a female talker. In each condition, there were 300 trials. On 90 of these trials, a target was presented, either to the right ear (45 trials) or to the left ear (45 trials). The remaining 210 trials were nontarget words in both conditions. By averaging evoked potentials separately for nontargets, and separately for right-ear targets and for left-ear targets in each condition, we were able to generate P300 waveforms separately for right and left ear targets in each condition, verbal and non-verbal. Results are summarized in Figure 4–4E. Note that the right ear pathway is intact for verbal targets, and the left ear pathway is

Procedure	RE	LE
Dichotic P300-Verbal Targets	OK	Absent
Dichotic P300-Non-Verbal Targets	Absent	OK

Figure 4–4E. Comparison of P300 event-related potential results for both verbal and nonverbal targets. Modified from Chmiel, R., Jerger, J., Murphy, E., Pirozzolo, F., and Tooley-Young C. (1997). Unsuccessful use of binaural amplification by an elderly person. *Journal of the American Academy of Audiology, 8*, 1–10.

intact for nonverbal pathways. The actual P300 waveforms are illustrated in Figure 4–4F at scalp electrode P3, where the greatest positive peak occurred. Note the positive peaks in the 600 to 1000-msec latency range. In the case of young adults, one would expect that the peak P300 voltages would be fairly similar for right and left ears, usually slightly greater for the right ear in the verbal condition, and slightly greater for the left ear for the nonverbal condition. In our participant, however, the P300 peak was robust for the right ear, but barely above the baseline for the left ear in the verbal condition. In the case of the nonverbal condition, the positive peak was robust for the left ear, but essentially absent for the right ear.

These results are best explained by a problem in transmission across the corpus callosal bridge. Consider the verbal condition; the right-ear targets travelled directly to the left hemisphere, were processed, and evoked a robust P300 peak, but the left-ear targets, required to follow the circuitous route, first to the right hemisphere, thence across the corpus callosum to the left hemisphere, evoked

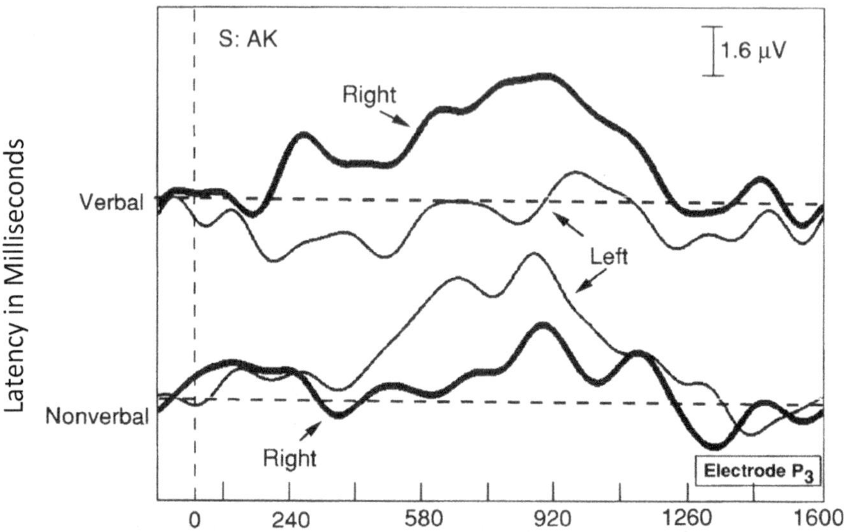

Figure 4–4F. Waveforms of P300 event-related potentials evoked by both verbal and nonverbal targets in dichotic paradigms. Modified from Chmiel, R., Jerger, J., Murphy, E., Pirozzolo, F., and Tooley-Young, C. (1997). Unsuccessful use of binaural amplification by an elderly person. *Journal of the American Academy of Audiology, 8,* 1–10.

little P300 response. On the other hand, in the nonverbal condition, the reverse was true. The left ear targets travelled directly to the right hemisphere, where they were successfully processed, while the right ear targets had to follow the circuitous route to the left hemisphere, then across the corpus callosum to the right hemisphere for processing as a nonverbal event. In this condition the P300 peak, although present, was also greatly attenuated.

Let us consider four possible alternative explanations for these unique findings:

1. Could it be a problem somewhere along the left-ear-to-right-hemisphere auditory pathway? Yes, that would easily explain the verbal condition, but no, it would hardly explain the robust P300 response to nonverbal targets.

2. Could it be a problem somewhere along the right-ear-to-left-hemisphere auditory pathway? No, that would hardly be consistent with the robust response to verbal targets.
3. Could it be a problem in the right auditory cortex? That would certainly explain the verbal target result, but would fail to explain the robust non-verbal target result.
4. Could it be a problem in the left auditory cortex? No, because although that would explain the nonverbal target result, it would fail to explain the robust verbal target result.

In short, only a problem in the bridge between the hemispheres can reasonably explain the P300 data. One take-home message here is that dichotic testing, supplemented by auditory event-related potentials, is a powerful tool for evaluating disorders of the central auditory system.

How does all this relate to binaural interference? Think about it this way. When the inputs from the two ears are not sufficiently similar, listening to speech processed simultaneously by the two ears is essentially a dichotic test with different verbal targets. If there is a callosal problem, the verbal input from the left ear will suffer degradation and perhaps interfere with the verbal input from the right ear. It is, perhaps, no accident that several investigators have commented that most of their cases of binaural interference seemed to favor the right ear over the left ear. The result is virtually forced by the fact that the test materials have been, uniformly, human speech.

SUMMARY

In this chapter, we describe, in some detail, audiometric findings in four cases in which there was clear evidence of binaural interference. Evidence ranged from better monaural than binaural speech recognition, to include, loss of the auditory brain stem response (ABR), loss of the auditory middle latency response (AMLR), and dichotic deficits revealed by P300 auditory event-related potentials (AERPs) to both verbal and nonverbal targets. One purpose in detailing these data has been to emphasize the importance of moving beyond simple speech recognition scores in order to establish solid documentation of binaural interference. A second purpose has been to show that, as data are gathered from carefully designed procedures, evidence mounts that the corpus callosum is a key structure in explaining the mechanism of some cases of binaural interference.

5

Clinical Evaluation of Binaural Interference

PREVIOUS HISTORY OF TESTING FOR BINAURAL INTERFERENCE

It is fair to say that, throughout the last five decades, the conditions under which binaural interference has been evaluated have varied widely. Table 5–1 summarizes testing conditions in the nine studies described in Chapter 1. Specific speech recognition tests varied widely across the nine studies: Two studies employed W-22 words, one study employed SSI Sentences, one study used VCV Syllables, two studies used QuickSIN, one study used Words in Noise (WIN), one study used HINT and the Connected Speech Test (CST), and one study used the Hebrew version of the AB open-set monosyllabic word test. For stimulus delivery, six studies employed sound-field testing, whereas the remaining three used headphones or insert receivers. In sound-field testing, the azimuth of the loudspeaker delivering the speech materials was always at 0°, but in the five studies presenting some form of competition during the speech testing, the competition source was at 180° in three studies, and at 0° in the remaining two studies. In the same five studies, the signal-to-competition ratio varied depending on the testing format. Across all nine studies, hearing aids were involved in four, and not in the other five. The presentation level of the speech materials varied according to the speech reception threshold (SRT) in two studies, at a fixed SPL in four studies, varied according to the test format in two studies, and at the most-comfortable loudness level (MCL) in one study.

Given the wide variety of conditions and parameters evident in Table 5–1, it would seem desirable to introduce some degree of standardization in testing for binaural interference. Here is a recommended approach.

Table 5–1. Testing Conditions in Nine Previous Studies of Binaural Interference

Study	Speech Recognition Test	Earphone or Sound Field?	Azimuth of Speech Speaker	Azimuth of Competition Speaker	S/N Ratio in dB	Hearing Aids?	Speech Presentation Level (dB)	Binaural Interference
Arkebauer et al. 1971	W-22 PB Words	Sound Field	0°	NA	NA	No	35 dB SL re SRT	80%
Jerger et al. 1993	SSI	Sound Field	0°	180°	–10 to +10	Yes	60 dB SPL	8%
Allen et al. 2000	W-22 PB Words	Insert Phones	NA	NA	NA	No	30 dB SL re SRT	0%
Karsten & Turner 2000	VCV Syllables	Insert Phones	NA	NA	NA	No	MCL	0%
Walden & Walden 2005	QuickSIN	Sound Field	0°	0°	+25 to 0	Yes	70 dB HL	82%
Henkin et al. 2007	Hebrew Words	Sound Field	0°	180°	+10	Yes	70 dB SPL	68%

continues

Table 5–1. *continued*

Study	Speech Recognition Test	Earphone or Sound Field?	Azimuth of Speech Speaker	Azimuth of Competition Speaker	S/N Ratio in dB	Hearing Aids?	Speech Presentation Level (dB)	Binaural Interference
Leigh-Paffenroth et al. 2011	Words In Noise (WIN)	Earphones	NA	NA	+24 to 0	No	Babble at 80 dB SPL Speech varied	0%
McArdle et al. 2012	QuickSIN	Sound Field	0°	0°	+25 to 0	Yes	70 dBHL	20%
Mussoi & Bentler 2017	HINT & CST	Sound Field	0°	180°	SNR-50	No	Noise at 65 dBA Speech varied	33%

Note. NA = Not Applicable.

CONFIGURATION OF TEST CHAMBER

Figure 5–1 shows a recommended arrangement for listener and loudspeaker placement. It is flexible to the extent that you can present the speech in three different configurations:

1. Speech but no competition
2. Speech and competition in the same speaker
3. Speech in front (0° azimuth) and competition from behind (180° azimuth).

All three arrangements have been employed in previous binaural interference studies. The third configuration is preferred for two

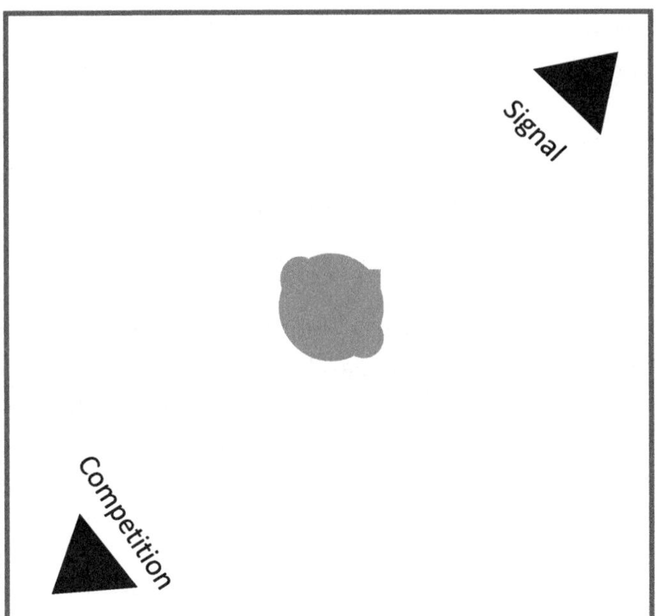

Figure 5–1. Our recommended arrangement for listener and loudspeaker placement.

reasons. First, it provides a source of competition that increases the difficulty of the listening task. Second, the source of competition is spatially separated from the speech source.

A TWO-STAGE APPROACH

It is useful to view testing for binaural interference as a two-stage process.

Screening

The first stage should be considered a screening procedure. The objective is simply to discover those individuals whose results suggest the need for further testing. We believe that, in the evaluation of adults, the screening measures of choice should be tests of speech recognition in a sound field under three conditions:

1. Binaural (both ears open)
2. Monaural Right Ear (left ear plugged)
3. Monaural Left Ear (right ear plugged)

Two commercially available tests of speech recognition have proven useful in previous research: (1) HINT, and (2) QuickSIN. One or the other of these two tests is recommended. Both are variations on adaptive procedures. In the HINT test, broadband noise spectrally matched to the speech is presented at a fixed level, whereas the speech materials are varied adaptively. In the QuickSIN procedure, speech is presented at a fixed level, and the level of four-talker babble is varied adaptively. In both procedures, the final score is a signal-to-competition ratio (commonly written as SNR) in dB. This metric is preferred over percentage correct scores for a variety of reasons (Leek, 2001; Levitt, 1971).

It is also important to emphasize the critical role of some form of competition in the speech recognition screening procedure. Testing speech recognition without competition has generally failed to be efficacious in revealing binaural interference (e.g., Carter, Noe, & Wilson, 2001).

Equally important is the need for testing in the sound field rather than via headphones or insert receivers. Given that researchers have yet to explore the effect of variation in azimuth of the speech speaker and azimuth of the competition speaker, the protocol should be based on azimuths investigated in previous binaural interference studies. That is, there should be two separate loudspeakers in the test chamber, one at 0° azimuth, to deliver the speech materials, the other at 180° azimuth, to deliver the competition. The presentation level should be 30 to 40 dB SL re SRT, separately determined for each of the three test conditions.

It bears repeating that the purpose of screening is simply to identify those individuals who need to be followed up with more intensive testing. Because the role of screening is to *not-miss-anybody* with a potential problem, a reasonable number of false positives can be tolerated. It might not be amiss to suggest that anyone whose best monaural score exceeds the binaural score by any amount has failed the screen.

It should also be emphasized that all of the above should be accomplished in the unaided condition. The introduction of amplification introduces more problems than are needed in a screening procedure. However, if the follow-up to a failed screen reveals evidence of a genuine problem in binaural interference, further evaluation with amplification can be carried out if desired, particularly when the use of amplification is being considered. Some of the problems you will face are discussed in a later section of this chapter.

We doubt that this arrangement for screening is optimal, and suggest other approaches in the next chapter. However, much work remains to be done on them before they can be recommended for general use.

Follow-Up Testing

If an individual fails the screen, follow-up testing should include: first a careful history of the client's chief complaint with special attention to any observed difference between the two ears; second, administration of a series of basic audiometric tests, followed by a series of site-specific tests:

Basic Audiometric Test Battery

The purpose of this sequence of basic tests is to paint a full picture of the extent and nature of the hearing loss, against which to evaluate the subsequent site-specific test results. It should include:

1. Pure-tone audiometry by air and bone conduction
2. Performance versus intensity (PI) functions for PB words: right ear, left ear, and binaural presentation.
3. Tympanometry and acoustic reflex (middle ear muscle) testing

Site-Specific Test Battery

Table 5–2 lists a series of site-specific tests we have found useful in documenting suspected binaural interference. The purpose of this sequence of tests is to identify any electrophysiological correlates of binaural interference, and to show the scope of binaural interference by demonstrating the various sites affected within the auditory system. As with speech testing, binaural interference would be evidenced by clearly better results on one of the monaural results, in comparison with the binaural result. The battery should include as many of the tests listed in Table 5–2 as possible or feasible.

The diagnosis of binaural interference can be entertained if there is at least one, but preferably two, confirmatory tests among those listed below. The absence of an electrophysiological finding

Table 5–2. Site-Specific Tests and their Known or Probable Sites in the Auditory System

Test	Wave	Latency in ms	Site
OAE			Cochlea—Outer Hair Cells
MEMR			Brain Stem—Ventral Cochlear Nucleus
ABR	I	1.7 ms	Cochlea—Spiral Ganglion
	III	3.8 ms	Brain Stem—Cochlear Nucleus
	V	5.7 ms	Brain Stem—Lateral Lemniscus?
AMLR	Pa	28 ms	Cortex—Synaptic Activation of cortex in core and belt regions
ALVR	N1b	100 ms	Auditory Cortex—Activation of widespread regions

Note. OAE = Otoacoustic Emissions; MEMR = Middle Ear Muscle Reflexes; ABR = Auditory Brain Stem Response; AMLR = Auditory Middle Latency Response; ALVR = Auditory Late Vertex Response; ms = milliseconds.

Source: Adapted and modified after Picton 2011, *Human Auditory Evoked Potentials,* p. 117.

of binaural interference may point to the need for monitoring of the patient to identify any subsequent emergence of a positive electrophysiological test result.

History

The audiologist should not only identify and quantify binaural interference, but also establish the impact of binaural interference on everyday life. The history should include questions on listening effort in challenging listening situations (e.g., in noise, group situations, reverberant environments), hearing aid preference/satisfaction and experience (e.g., if fitted binaurally but prefer a monaural fitting), and localization. Noble, Jensen, Naylor, Bhullar, and Akeroyd (2013) developed a short form of the Speech, Spatial, and Qualities of Hearing Scale (SSQ12) that contains 12 items that sample speech in noise, multiple speech streams, speech in speech, localization, distance, and movement (e.g., "Can you tell how far away a bus or a truck is from the sound?"), segregation (e.g., "When you hear more than one sound at a time, do you have the impression that it seems like single jumbled sound?"), identification of sound, quality, and naturalness, listening effort. This questionnaire can easily be incorporated into the audiological history-taking process.

SOME ISSUES RELATING TO TESTING WITH HEARING AIDS

Although binaural interference and hearing aids have become interwoven in the real world, it is important to remember that binaural interference is a separate concept, independent of hearing aids. It has been demonstrated via headphones, insert receivers, and sound field testing without providing any external amplification for the two ears. If, however, the issue of amplification is to be pursued, here are some additional problems.

First, there is the question of how the gains of the aids are to be set. In some studies, the two gains have been adjusted according to a formula (e.g., NAL). In other studies, the gain of each aid is separately set to comfort level, and these settings remain in the binaural condition. Both of these approaches have been criticized because the settings based on monaural listening may be excessively loud in the binaural condition. In still other studies, the user has reset the gains of both aids in the binaural condition. At present, there is no known standard procedure dealing with gain settings for aided speech-in-noise testing. A related issue is the presentation level and hearing aid gain/maximum levels. Excessively high levels can yield hearing aid distortion that can adversely influence performance on binaural interference tests. Lastly, differences in hearing aid signal processing (e.g., digital processing delay differences) in the binaural condition might influence performance on binaural interference tests (Mussoi & Bentler, 2017). This series of issues is so complex that we hesitate to offer specific advice until all have had the benefit of further systematic research. In the meantime, caution is advised whenever attempting to evaluate binaural interference in the presence of amplification.

Second, there is the issue of whether to plug the nontest ear in monaural testing, to guard against inflating the best monaural score due to the possible contribution of the open nontest ear to the monaural score of the test ear (McArdle, Killion, Mennite, & Chisolm, 2012). The problem here is that plugging the nontest ear is, itself, an unnatural condition. The monaural hearing aid user does not ordinarily go through life with the nonfitted ear plugged. Apparently, most investigators have removed the hearing aid from the nontest ear during monaural testing in order to duplicate the real life situation (details on this issue are not always given in the methods sections of articles). This may be the preferred procedure for evaluating how one versus two hearing aids will actually work for the individual in everyday life.

SUMMARY

A review of nine previous studies of binaural interference shows little uniformity in procedural details, suggesting that it might be desirable to seek a somewhat more standardized approach to the diagnosis of binaural interference. We outline a two-staged approach: (1) a screening procedure involving speech recognition testing in the sound field, followed by, (2) a more intensive follow-up, employing site specific diagnostic tests to either confirm or deny the screening outcome. All of this is carried out without amplification. If further testing with hearing aids is desired, the reader is cautioned about additional problems likely to be encountered.

Research is needed to investigate different remediation strategies when binaural interference is detected. In an individual with bilateral, symmetric sensorineural hearing loss, for example, who is binaurally aided, remediation might not always necessitate a change in fitting from binaural to monaural. The case study presented by Boothroyd (1993) demonstrates that binaural fitting can be accomplished after rejection of binaural amplification in some circumstances. Should auditory training attempt to strengthen the weak ear and/or should it promote the strength of the already dominant ear? These are all issues that need to be sorted out.

6

Future Directions

In this chapter, we consider what the future may hold for binaural interference testing. Are there better ways to detect and evaluate it? Binaural interference is usually defined by the fact that a monaural speech recognition score is better than the corresponding binaural score. However, because there is always error of measurement, we would like the difference between the two scores to be large relative to error. One way to approach this issue is to ask how well the proposed technique detects a binaural advantage in people not suspected of binaural interference. There has been voluminous literature over many years documenting the theoretical and objectively demonstrated advantages of binaural over monaural hearing. If a test procedure cannot reveal this advantage in a normal listener, how confident can we be that it will reveal the opposite effect in a person suspected of binaural interference? Clearly, the first step in the search for a better test of binaural interference is to ask how well it can detect a binaural advantage when it ought to be there. Interestingly, none of the nine studies summarized in Table 5–1 reported data bearing on this question. In the following sections, we ask what is the best way to measure binaural advantage in normal listeners and in persons with hearing loss. Are traditional speech recognition tests sufficient, or is there a better way to approach the problem?

WHAT IS THE BEST WAY TO MEASURE BINAURAL ADVANTAGE?

Why do we have two ears? What is the evolutionary advantage? Writers on binaural hearing often cite, as a vivid example of the value of the binaural system, the "cocktail party effect" (the ability to focus on a specific voice from amid myriad voices and a general background of sonic competition). But the evolutionary importance of this phenomenon is not obvious.

If you are an animal in the wild, your two principal concerns are to eat and to not be eaten. It is vital, therefore, that you have a sense of the surrounding space and the direction from which a predator, or prey, approaches or flees. These two dimensions, space and directionality, define the essential evolutionary significance of the two-eared system (Møller, 2000). It follows that if you want to study the binaural advantage (or disadvantage), the places to look are auditory space and directionality. Of the two, directionality would seem to be a more practical candidate for our purposes.

Importance of Directionality

Figure 6–1 shows the currently popular arrangement for testing speech recognition in the sound field. The listener faces the source of the test words or sentences at 0° azimuth. There may

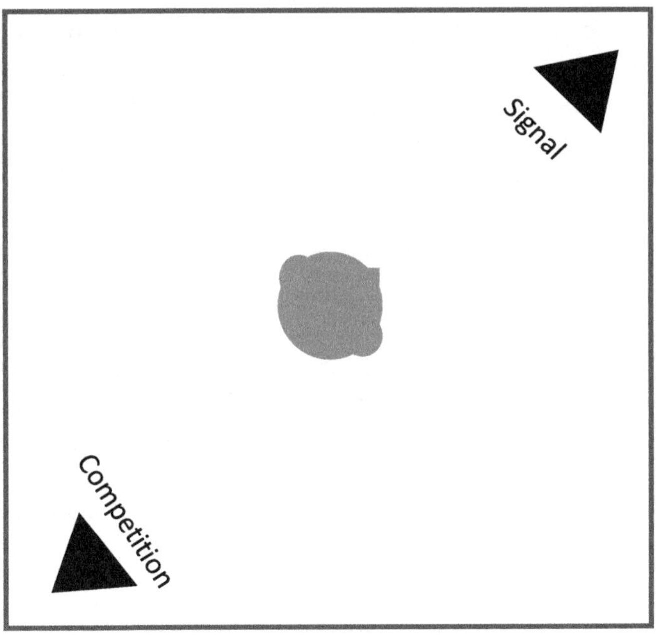

Figure 6–1. Arrangement of listener and loudspeakers in traditional sound-field speech audiometric testing.

or may not be some form of competition, either from the same loudspeaker at 0° azimuth or directly behind the listener at 180° azimuth. Now, as noted in Chapter 5, Figure 5–1, this has been the basic configuration in many of the recent studies searching for the prevalence of binaural interference. However, it is hardly the best arrangement for demonstrating the directionality dimension afforded by the two-eared system. It would be surprising indeed if there were large differences among results for left ear alone, right ear alone, and binaural alone, or their aided counterparts. Although all of the authors of the studies summarized in Figure 5–1 asked the question, "Was there binaural interference?" none appear to have asked the counter question, "Was my methodology capable of showing a significant binaural advantage?" It is perhaps axiomatic that a procedure incapable of demonstrating that two ears are better than one may also be incapable of demonstrating that two ears are worse than one.

How can we study the ability to tell the direction from which a word or sentence is sourced? The most straightforward solution is to eschew the one-loudspeaker arrangement involving a loudspeaker at 0° azimuth in favor of a two-speaker arrangement in which one loudspeaker is located to the right of the listener and the other loudspeaker is located an equal distance to the left of the listener. One possible arrangement is illustrated in Figure 6–2. In this example, the left loudspeaker is located at 15° azimuth from midline, the other at 345° azimuth In other words, each loudspeaker is offset 15° from the midline, yielding a 30° angle between the two loudspeakers. A simple test procedure would be to present W-22 words from a loudspeaker chosen at random, with the constraint that each loudspeaker presents exactly 50% of the words. Instructions to the listener are: "Tell me what word you heard, then tell me which loudspeaker delivered the word?" From these responses, you can compute:

1. an overall W-22 score,
2. a separate W-22 score for the right loudspeaker,

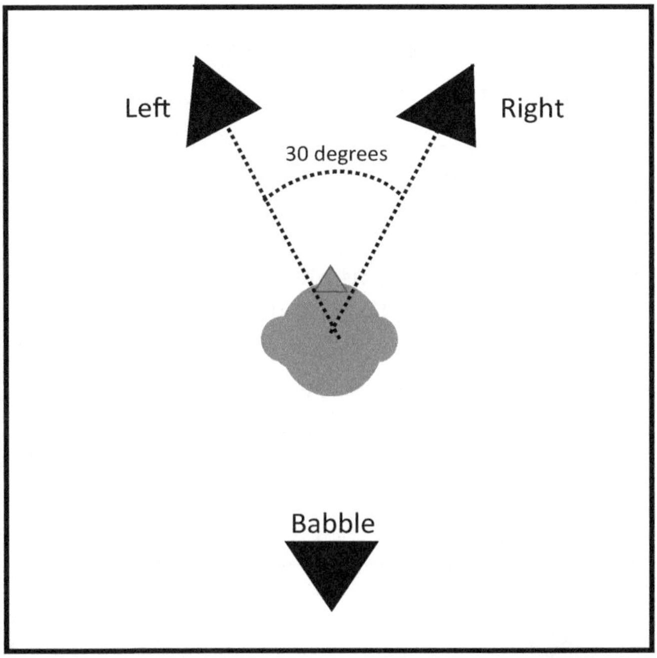

Figure 6–2. Another possible arrangement of loudspeakers speakers and listener, designed to capture data on directionality in the listening experience.

3. a separate W-22 score for the left loudspeaker,
4. an overall directional error score from the listeners second response in each trial,
5. a separate directional error score for the right loudspeaker.
6. a separate directional error score for the left loudspeaker.

The possible variations on this simple arrangement are countless. You can vary the angular distance between loudspeakers until normal listeners score at about 80% to 90%, and you can manipulate the task difficulty by making the signal-to-babble ratio more or less favorable for the listener. Once you have settled on the optimal parameters, you can proceed to test hearing-impaired persons in the three standard conditions: monaural right, monaural left, and binaural.

Cued Listening

If you really want to get serious about the search for quantifying binaural advantage and facilitating the detection of binaural disadvantage, you might want to consider cued listening. It is a bit more complicated and takes somewhat more testing time, but the results are worth the additional effort. Figure 6–3 shows a design developed some years ago at the Baylor College of Medicine

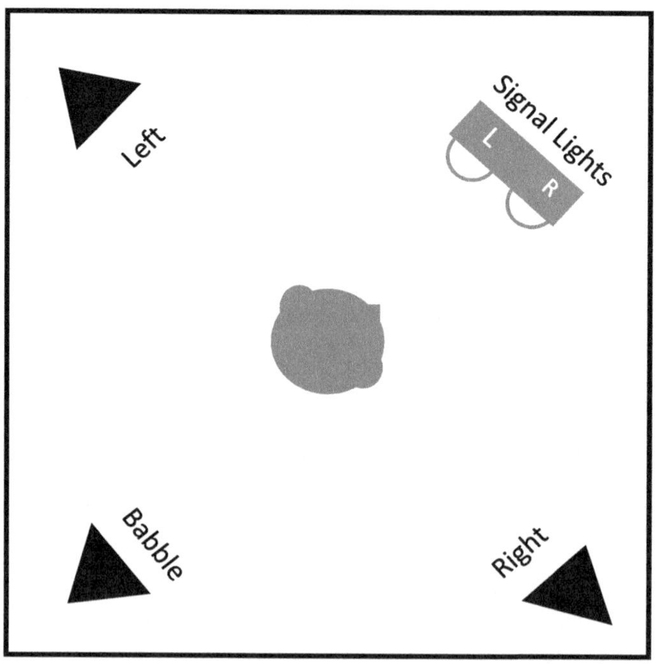

Figure 6–3. An even more directionality-oriented arrangement—cued listening.

(Jerger & Jordan, 1992). Again there are two loudspeakers, but now they are located at 90° azimuth (directly opposite the right ear) and at 270° azimuth (directly opposite the left ear). In other words, the angular separation between loudspeakers is now 180°. The auditory stimulus is a section of running speech. An excerpt from any interesting story will due as long as a simple repetitive phonological target is available. Jerger and Jordan used the pronoun "I" in a detective story written in the first-person singular (e.g., *"I got up and had some breakfast. Then I strapped on my holster, but I couldn't find my gun . . . "* etc.). This story segment is delivered by both loudspeakers but the story is offset by 60 seconds in one loudspeaker relative to the other. Thus, the listener hears the same story from each loudspeaker, but it is always a slightly different part of the story from each side. The idea here is that we are no longer interested in a speech recognition score, in itself. We are using the running speech only as a medium in which to imbed a phonological target that is being presented from both sides of auditory space, but in an altered, temporal position due to the time delay between the stories on the two sides. Our principal interest is in two measures: (1) correct identifications; how well does the listener respond to targets presented from the precued side of space, and (2) directional errors; how often does the listener false alarm in relation to correct directional responses to the precued side as a proportion of correct responses.

A total of 100 targets are presented, 50 from the right side and 50 from the left side. The side to be attended is signaled by one of the two lights, labeled "Listen Right" and "Listen Left" on the console directly facing the listener. The side to be attended is signaled in five blocks of 10 "I"s from each side, with the constraint that no target loudspeaker is cued more than twice in succession. A loudspeaker located directly behind the listener delivers multitalker babble whose level can be adjusted to achieve the degree of desired difficulty of the listening task.

The listener has two response buttons, one held in the right hand, the other in the left hand. The task is simply to press the appropriate response button whenever an "I" is heard, but it must be an "I" from the side cued by the signal light. If such response occurs within 1.5 seconds of the onset of the "I," this is scored as a correct identification. Failure to respond to a presented "I" within the acceptable time frame is considered a miss. The number of misses for a particular side is calculated by subtracting the number of correct identifications from 50. If, however, the listener responded by pressing the response button to any "I" presented from the wrong side within the 1.5-second response window, that response was considered a laterality error. Laterality errors are especially relevant to the specific dimension of directionality.

Jerger and Jordan (1992) published cued-listening results for 10 young adults with normal hearing and 28 elderly persons with high-frequency presbyacusic-like audiometric configurations. They presented the story level at each listener's comfort level and varied the MCR from 0 to −15 dB. In the young adult group, the right ear advantage for correct identification scores [(R − L)/ (R + L), averaged across the 4 MCR conditions] was 2.4%. In the elderly group, the comparable average value was 15.8%, but the variability among elderly participants was much greater, a left ear disadvantage exceeding 40% in many members of the elderly group.

Further data from this study included results of aided scores in two elderly hearing-aid users. The first, a 67-year-old woman, reported that her binaural aids were helpful in difficult listening situations. She was a satisfied binaural user. Her PTAs were 32 dB on the right ear and 42 dB on the left ear. The PB scores were 84% on the right ear and 64% on the left ear. On the cued-listening test, her best monaural aided score, averaged across target right and target left conditions, was 52%, and her binaural aided score, averaged across target right and target left conditions, was 78%, yielding a binaural advantage of 26%. In contrast, the second elderly binaural aid user, a 68-year-old woman, reported that her aids did not help in most listening situations. She was unhappy with them. Her PTAs were 40 dB on the right ear and 33 dB on the left ear. The PB scores were 84% on both ears. On the cued-listening test, the aided left ear score, collapsed across target condition, was 30%, the binaural aided score, was 6%, a binaural disadvantage of 24%.

Here then were two experienced binaural hearing aid users: comparable ages, same gender, comparable degree of loss and comparable unaided PB scores. The satisfied user showed a binaural advantage of 26%, the unhappy user a binaural disadvantage of 24%.

In a later paper (Jerger, Darling, & Florin, 1994), the authors employed the cued listening task to evaluate the performance of 10 experienced and entirely satisfied binaural aid users. Again, the rationale was that a technique incapable of demonstrating a binaural advantage when it was expected might not be very effective at detecting binaural interference. Conversely, a technique capable of showing a robust binaural advantage, might reflect robust binaural interference as well.

The MCR was fixed at 0 dB. Figure 6–4A shows the cued listening results, averaged across the 10 listeners over four conditions; unaided, aided left, aided right, and aided binaural. If you want to find actual data confirming that binaural aids can be advantageous, the cued listening task is a procedure that seems especially efficacious. The average difference between the aided-right score and the aided binaural score across the ten participants was a robust 19.7%. Of the ten participants, all showed best performance in the binaural-aided condition, a not unexpected finding because they had been pre-selected because they were experienced and satisfied users of binaural aids. However, the actual individual binaural advantage scores varied substantially. Of the ten individual difference scores between best monaural and binaural results, all 10 showed a better binaural score than either monaural score. Seven were statistically significant at the 5% level by the nonparametric randomization test for single-subject data (Edgington, 1967). Figures 6–4B and 6–4C show illustrative findings in two individual members of the group.

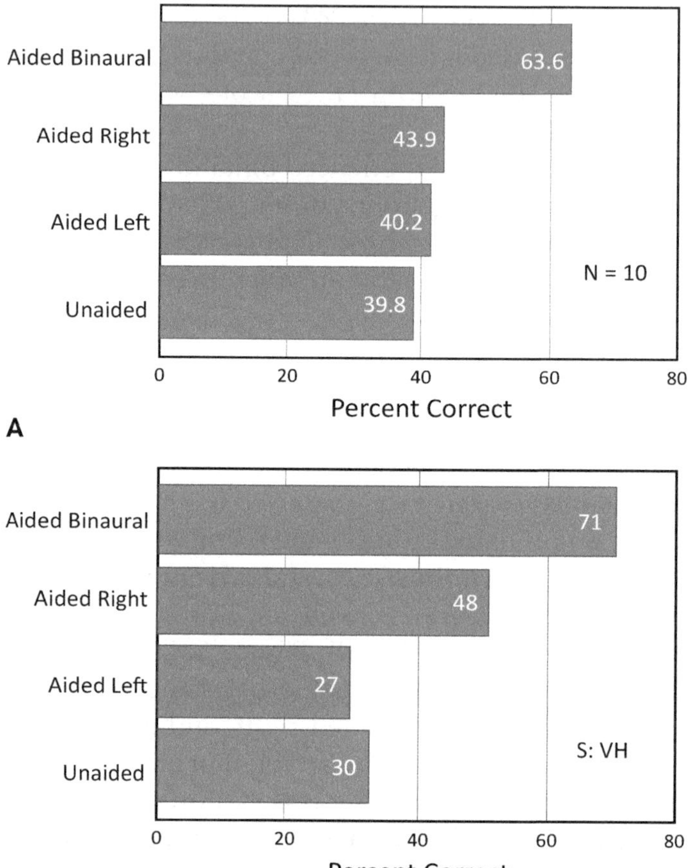

A

B

Figure 6–4. A. Average cued-listening results across 10 experienced and satisfied binaural hearing aid users. Note substantial binaural advantage compared to right ear alone. **B.** Largest binaural advantage recorded among the 10 listeners whose average cued-listening results are displayed in **A**.

Participant VH (Figure 6–4B) had the largest binaural advantage, a difference of 23% between the best monaural aided score and the binaural aided score. Not unexpectedly, VH also showed the

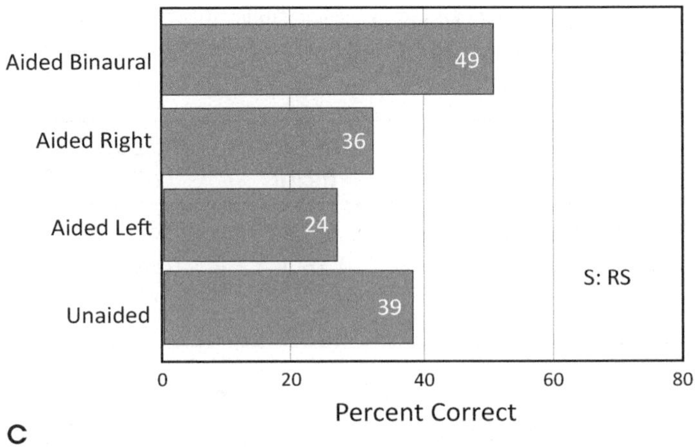

Figure 6–4. *continued* **C.** Smallest binaural advantage recorded among the 10 listeners whose average cued-listening results are displayed in **A**.

largest difference between the unaided score and the binaural aided score (41%). Participant RS (Figure 6–4C), on the other hand, had the smallest binaural advantage (13%), but the binaural aided score was still 10% better than the unaided score. It is also noteworthy that the aided-right score was better than the aided-left score in every one of the ten participants. In the case of VH, the difference was an astonishing 21%.

What happens to this robust binaural advantage on the cued listening test in the person with documented binaural interference? Consider Case #3 from Chapter 4. This was the 81-year-old man with compelling evidence of binaural interference in the AMLR evoked potentials. His cued listening data are summarized in Table 6–1. Up to this point, we have presented only cued listening data on correct identifications, but a second measure, laterality error, was recorded whenever the listener incorrectly responded to an "I" from the wrong direction. We have, then, for each of the three aided conditions, both correct identifications and laterality errors. The data of Case #3 (see Table 6–1) show

Table 6–1. Comparison of Correct Identifications (CI), Laterality Errors (LE), and CI/LE Ratios Derived from the Cued-Listening Data of Case # 3 in Chapter 4

	Aided Right	Aided Left	Aided Binaural
Correct Identifications (CI)	37%	18%	34%
Laterality Errors (LE)	17%	15%	28%
CI/LE	2.2	1.2	1.2

that, in the aided right condition, the correct identification rate was 37%, the laterality error rate 17%, yielding a correct identification-to-laterality ratio of 2.2. In the aided left ear condition, the ratio was only 1.2. And, not unexpectedly, the ratio for the binaural aided condition was a similar 1.2. When the laterality error rate almost equals the correct identification rate, the binaural aids are not doing a very good job for the listener.

The crucial point here is that laterality errors are directional errors. And, in a system specialized for directional accuracy, directional errors are unfortunate. This is the feature of everyday life in which the two-eared system ought to excel. The cued-listening task seems particularly sensitive to capturing errors in this important dimension of two-eared hearing.

It is certainly the case that the cued-listening task is cognitively demanding, especially for elderly persons, but the demand is similar for targets coming from either direction.

In Search of a Pitch Mismatch and Abnormal Binaural Fusion

Reiss, Eggleston, Walker, and Oh (2016) hypothesized that abnormal binaural spectral integration might underlie the binaural interference demonstrated with the vowel classification patterns by some binaural hearing-aid users. They suggested that:

> In the hearing-impaired auditory system, however, the two ears are often mismatched in pitch, leading to an incongruency of spectral information between ears. If incongruent spectral information is fused and averaged between ears, different percepts may underlie binaural as compared to monaural stimulation. . . . Can abnormal binaural integration account for reduced speech perception benefit, or even interference, with two ears compared to one? (p. 342)

For the interaural pitch and fusion range studies on a subset of the users of hearing aids, interaural pitch matching was based on a two-interval, two-alternative, forced-choice, constant-stimulus procedure. A reference tone was presented to one ear and a comparison tone of a different frequency was presented to the opposite ear. Loudness balance was accomplished across all tone frequencies. The listener's task was to identify the ear that heard the higher-pitched tone. Frequency spacing between the reference and comparison tones was accomplished by varying the frequency of the comparison tone in 1/4-octave steps within the residual hearing frequency range, while holding the reference frequency constant. Because there were at least six trials at each frequency, a psychometric function was constructed showing, for each reference tone, the average percent of time the comparison tone was judged to be higher in pitch than the reference tone. The pitch match frequency was that associated with the 50% point on the psychometric function. The magnitude of the interaural pitch mismatch can then be computed. Figures 6–5 and 6–6 illustrate the experimental design and schematic of a sample psychometric function, respectively for pitch matching. Figure 6–6 illustrates the subject's response options during a single trial.

The investigators observed, for their hearing-aid users, that interaural pitch mismatches were larger at the F1 frequencies

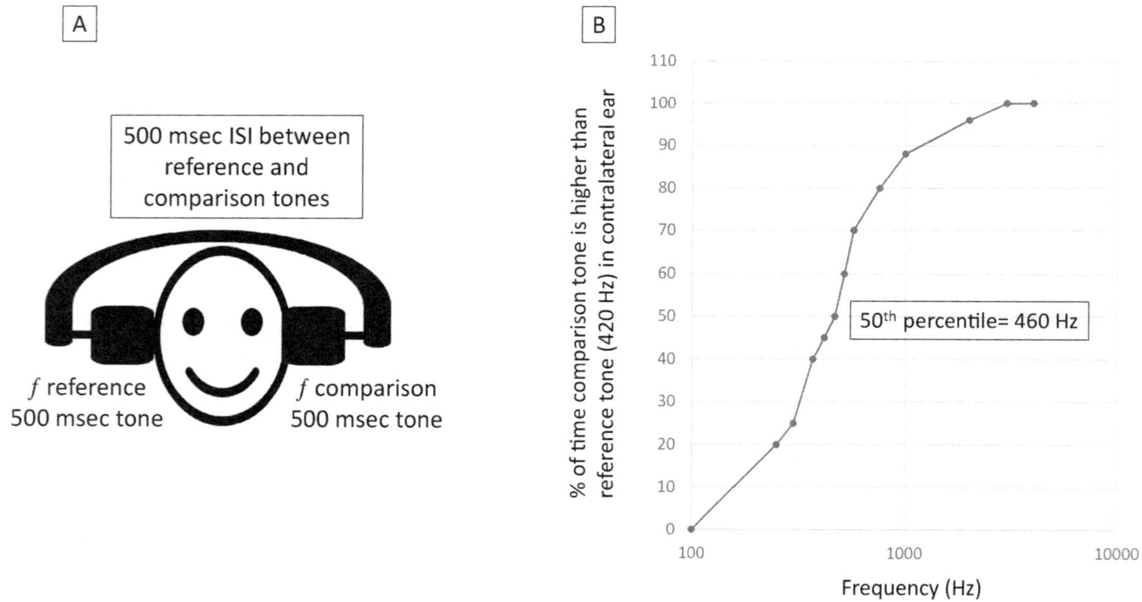

Figure 6–5. A. shows the setup for the interaural pitch match experiment. The tone in the reference ear is fixed and the comparison tone in the contralateral ear is varied in 1/4 octave steps between 125 and 4000 Hz. The interstimulus interval (ISI) between the reference and comparison tones is 500 msec. The participant's task was to select the ear that received the higher pitched tone. **B.** Shows a schematic of the psychometric function based on the averaging of responses (each frequency was repeated six times) at each frequency. The pitch match represents the 50th percentile on the psychometric function. In this schematic, the reference tone is 420 Hz and the 50th percentile for the interaural pitch match occurs at 460 Hz.

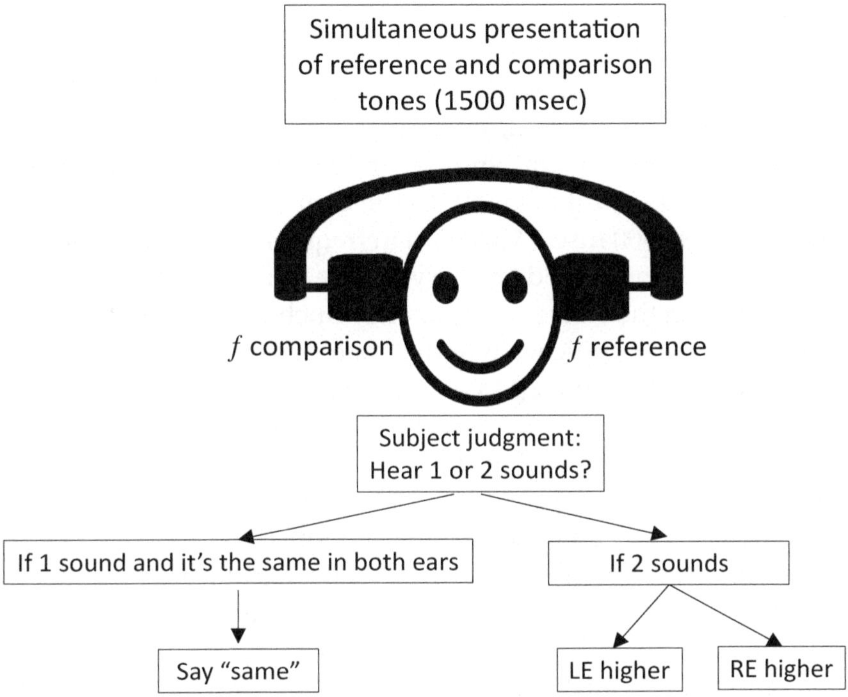

Figure 6–6. The setup for fusion range measurement. The reference and comparison tones are delivered simultaneously (rather than sequentially as in the interaural pitch match experiment). The fusion range represents the frequency range within which a single tone is heard at least 50% of the time.

when binaural interference was seen on synthetic vowel classification patterns than when the classification patterns did not demonstrate binaural interference. The range of interaural pitch mismatches for vowel classification patterns associated with binaural interference on synthetic vowels in the small sample of users of hearing aids who could be tested with this procedure was 717 to 872 Hz; the range of interaural pitch mismatches for the patterns not associated with binaural interference was 388 to 777 Hz.

For measurement of fusion range, that is, the frequency range over which dichotic tones are fused and heard as a single tone rather than as two tones, Reiss et al. (2016) employed a forced-choice task. At each trial, one frequency (reference tone) was presented to one ear and another frequency (comparison tone) was presented simultaneously to the contralateral ear. Stimulus duration was 1500 msec. Variation in frequency separation across trials was accomplished by varying the comparison frequency while keeping the reference frequency unchanged. The listener's task was to first indicate whether one or two tones were perceived. If one tone was perceived, then the listener was to say "same." If two tones were perceived, then the listener specified the ear in which the higher frequency tone was perceived. The fusion range was computed to be the frequency range across trials in which the listener perceived only one tone (said, "same"). They observed, for their hearing aid users, that fusion ranges were broader for binaural interference synthetic vowel patterns than for other synthetic vowel patterns. The results for their small sample revealed the fusion range to be 1.7 to 2.8 octaves for binaural interference patterns, and 0.2 to 2.4 octaves for vowel classification patterns not associated with binaural interference. This finding was corroborated by Reiss et al. (2017) on a larger sample; the mean fusion range was 1.7 octaves in their group of 16 listeners with varying degrees of bilateral, sensorineural hearing loss (14 were users of bilateral hearing aids), as compared with a much smaller mean fusion range of 0.17 octave in their group of 10 normal-hearing listeners. Similar findings were obtained by Oh and Reiss (2017) for their group of bimodal cochlear implant users and for their group of bilateral hearing aid users.

SUMMARY

We have argued in this chapter that given the evolutionary importance of having two ears to determine the direction from which sound is coming, auditory tests of binaural interference should explore the dimension of directionality. Auditory measures that are insensitive to the presence of binaural advantage also might be insensitive to the presence of binaural interference/binaural disadvantage.

The simplest approach described for exploring binaural interference, based on directionality dimension, involves a two-speaker arrangement in the sound field. The angle between speakers can be varied over a 180° range . Speech-in-babble noise (at any signal-to-babble ratio) can be presented through one loudspeaker (right versus left at random). The listener is tasked to identify the stimulus and then to identify the loudspeaker that delivered the stimulus. Speech-recognition scores can be calculated (total score across loudspeakers, score for right loudspeaker, score for left loudspeaker). Additionally, direction and location error scores can be calculated (total directional error score across loudspeakers, location error score for the right loudspeaker, and location error score for the left loudspeaker). These scores can be obtained in the aided or unaided monaural right, monaural left, and binaural conditions.

A more sophisticated approach described, that may yield more dividends for evaluating binaural advantage and disadvantage, is based on the Jerger and Jordan (1992) cued-listening design and the modifications by Jerger, Darling, and Florin (1994). Here, the same story is presented through two loudspeakers on each side of the listener, but the story on one side is offset by 1 minute relative to the same story on the opposite side. Two lights ("right" and "left") in front of the listener cue the listener to the loudspeaker (right or left) to be attended when listening to the story to detect instances where "I" (or other target) is heard on the side cued. The listener is instructed to press a response button (right or left) associated with the side on which the target was heard. Both monaural aided scores, and the binaural aided scores, can be obtained based on the percentage correct identification of the loudspeaker side during target delivery. Comparison of these scores enables detection and quantification of binaural advantage and disadvantage. In each condition (e.g., aided right, aided left, and binaural), the ratio of correct identifications ("hits") to laterality errors (false alarms) can be computed. A three-pronged approach can be taken to quantify binaural advantage and disadvantage: (a) by comparing correct identifications across the three aided conditions; (b) by comparing laterality errors across conditions; and (c) by comparing the laterality error rate in the binaural aided condition with the hit rate in the same condition.

Both approaches have been applied for the study of binaural advantage and disadvantage/interference. Results show the approaches are feasible and efficacious. Additionally, these procedures appear to corroborate hearing aid use complaints/dissatisfaction. These procedures also lend themselves to a myriad of variations on the design, such as angular separation between speakers, speech material, speech-to-babble ratio, and offset time.

Interaural pitch matching and fusion range procedures represent psychoacoustical perspectives for evaluating binaural interference. Both procedures involve a reference tone presented to one ear and a comparison tone presented to the other ear. The procedure for interaural pitch matching involves an interstimulus interval between the tones, whereas the procedure for fusion range involves simultaneous presentation of the tones. With the interaural pitch matching procedure, the frequency spacing is varied, and the listener is instructed to state the ear in which the higher frequency is heard. The pitch match frequency associated with 50% on the psychometric function is computed. For the fusion procedure, the frequency range over which the listeners judges the reference and frequency tones to be the same/fused is established. The idea is that the large interaural pitch mismatches and broad binaural fusion may be associated with binaural interference. These psychoacoustical procedures need validation on larger samples so that feasibility and efficacy can be established.

7
Overview

LESSONS LEARNED

1. Binaural Interference is, at present, a phenomenon unique to speech understanding. It is perhaps best conceptualized as interaural rivalry. A weakened ear, usually the left ear, appears to be dominated by the stronger ear. As a result, speech is not understood as well when both ears are stimulated simultaneously, as when only the stronger ear is stimulated.
2. Although binaural interference necessarily impacts the successful use of binaural hearing aids, it exists as an abnormality in the auditory system, independent of amplification. Much of the literature on binaural interference has focused on aided speech understanding scores across the three conditions of monaural right, monaural left, and binaural, often in the aided condition. However, the phenomenon has been observed in the ABR, the AMLR, dichotic listening tests, and the P300 auditory event-related potential, and in pitch matching.
3. Estimates of the prevalence of binaural interference have varied widely, depending on the test methodology employed, and the age range of the cohort studied. Three generalizations however seem warranted: (a) It appears to be most frequent among elderly hearing-impaired persons; (b) Best estimates of prevalence are about 10% to 20% of the elderly hearing-impaired population; and (c) It seems unrelated to the degree of sensorineural hearing loss.
4. Quite a few elderly hearing aid users seem to prefer one hearing aid over two. In retrospective studies, the percentage preferring one aid increased from 3% to 31% between 1981 and 2009. In field trials, the percentage has ranged from 7% to an astonishing 61% over that same time frame. It is certainly the case that there are reasons other than binaural interference for preferring only one aid in surveys and field trials, but at least some must surely be attributed to binaural interference.

5. At least three different bases for binaural interference have been identified in hearing-impaired persons: (a) prolonged auditory deprivation; (b) age-related changes in the corpus callosum; and (c) abnormal binaural fusion of sounds between the two ears.
6. Case studies have advanced our understanding of binaural interference by showing how a test battery approach can identify binaural interference unequivocally, and can sometimes isolate the level of abnormality along the auditory pathways from ear to cortex.
7. Testing only the right aided, left aided, and binaurally aided conditions represents a minimal approach to detection of binaural interference and contributes little to understanding the levels of the auditory system affected by the problem, the scope of the problem, and the impact of the problem in everyday life.
8. The traditional approach to the evaluation of binaural interference—presentation of speech test materials from a loudspeaker directly in front of the listener, at 0° azimuth—is probably not the best approach. Techniques based on measuring the accuracy of directionality judgements are more desirable.

SUMMARY OF THE BOOK

Chapter 1 briefly summarized the history of the phenomenon of binaural interference. Nearly 80 years ago, Vern Knudsen of UCLA predicted that, when binaural hearing aids became a reality, some individuals with sensorineural hearing loss who experienced interaural pitch discrepancy (diplacusis) might have unsatisfactory experiences (interaural conflict) with binaural hearing-aids. Further exploration into interaural conflict did not occur until 1971, when Arkebauer, Mencher, and McCall observed that, in individuals with asymmetric sensorineural hearing loss, word-recognition scores in sound field were better in the monaural (poorer ear occluded) condition than in the binaural condition (poorer ear unoccluded) in 8 of 10 participants. In 1984, Silman, Gelfand, and Silverman reported that speech-recognition scores can decline significantly over time in the unaided ear of monaurally fitted individuals with bilateral, symmetric sensorineural hearing loss, whose pure-tone sensitivity does not decline over time, This phenomenon, termed auditory deprivation, might possibly account for Arkebauer et al.'s finding.

The seminal report on binaural interference was published in 1993 by Jerger, Silman, Lew, and Chmiel. Their case studies, further described in Chapter 4, illustrated the phenomenon of binaural interference in both aided and unaided speech recognition scores and in diagnostic measures, including the ABR, the AMLR, dichotic tests, and the P300 auditory event-related potentials.

Silman's (1995) case study on a patient with multiple sclerosis is notable, not only for illustrating electrophysiological evidence of binaural interference on the auditory brainstem response (ABR), but also on the auditory middle latency response (AMLR).

Chapter 2 examined indirect evidence that binaural hearing is not always better than monaural hearing in individuals with bilateral, symmetric, sensorineural hearing loss. One line of evidence arose from a study by Rothpletz, Tharpe, and Grantham (2004) in which the effects of sensorineural hearing loss were simulated in three listening conditions: (a) monaural signal degradation, (b) binaural, symmetric signal degradation, and (c) binaural, asymmetric signal degradation. Findings in young, normal-hearing adults showed worse performance under the binaural, asymmetric signal degradation condition than under the binaural, symmetric signal degradation condition—evidence, indeed, that two ears are not always better than one. However, generalizing the findings from such studies to individuals with hearing loss is always problematic.

The second line of evidence came from retrospective surveys of hearing-aid users; the findings of these surveys indicate that preference for one hearing aid over two is not uncommon.

A study by Noble, Jensen, Naylor, Bhullar, and Akeroyd (2013) showed the feasibility of using a questionnaire that taps auditory spatial abilities when investigating binaural interference. For example, one item in the spatial category, "locate barking dog" clearly differentiated between the unilateral and bilateral hearing aid preference groups. The third line of evidence that binaural is not always better than monaural amplification came from structured field trials on preference for one versus two hearing aids. The percentage of individuals who preferred one hearing aid over two was even more pronounced (20% to 61%) with the field trials than with the retrospective studies. In one field trial (Cox, Schwartz, Noe, & Alexander, 2011), over 50% of the participants listed reasons for such preference such as "in noisy situations I understand speech as well or better when I wear only one hearing aid." Of course, the disadvantage of both retrospective and field trial studies is that reasons for preferring one to two hearing aids may reflect factors other than binaural interference.

Chapter 3 considered possible bases for binaural interference. We began with a review of the neuroanatomy of the auditory system from ear to brain, stressing, in particular, the prepotency of the crossed pathways from each ear to the contralateral hemisphere of the brain, coupled with the observation that in most right-handed individuals, speech input to either ear must be processed in the left hemisphere. The net effect, for most right-handed persons, is a slight advantage to right-ear input due to its privileged access to the speech processing centers in the left hemisphere. In order for speech input from the left-ear to be processed in the left hemisphere, it must travel from the right hemisphere to the left hemisphere via a neural bridge, the corpus callosum. This puts the left ear at a constant disadvantage, slight in young adults with normal hearing, but larger and larger as age-related changes affect the efficiency of transmission across the callosal bridge linking the two hemispheres.

Following this tutorial, we considered three possible bases for binaural interference: (1) auditory deprivation; (2) age-related declines in efficiency of interhemispheric transfer or in cortical inhibition; and (3) abnormal binaural fusion of sounds between the two ears.

The seminal study on auditory deprivation was reported by Silman, Gelfand, and Silverman (1984). The linkage between auditory deprivation and rejection of binaural amplification in favor of monaural amplification, suggestive of binaural interference, came from Hurley (1993), who observed that 4 of 9 participants with bilateral, symmetric, sensorineural hearing loss who were initially fitted monaurally and then were fitted binaurally years later after incurring auditory deprivation in the unaided ear, subsequently rejected binaural amplification. The linkage between auditory deprivation and binaural interference was further established by the finding (Wieselberg & Iório, 2012) of changes in the auditory cortex as evidenced by a prolonged mean P300 latency in the unaided ear, as compared with the aided ear of monaurally fitted adults.

The most recently advanced hypothesis for a cause of binaural interference, presented in Chapter 3, emerged from the study by Reiss, Eggleston, Walker, and Oh (2016). They examined vowel classification performance for pairs of synthetic vowels (differing in F1 values, yet essentially similar in F2 values) in each monaurally aided condition and in the binaurally aided condition, and observed, in some of the binaurally fitted hearing-aid users, patterns indicative of binaural interference, such as a binaural vowel classification pattern falling in between the two monaural vowel classification patterns, and a binaural vowel classification pattern differing from both monaural patterns, with poorer speech-recognition than either monaural pattern. They observed abnormally broad fusion of sounds presented simultaneously to the two ears in the hearing-aid users who displayed binaural interference on the vowel classification patterns.

In Chapter 4, presentation of four case studies furnished a framework for understanding the various manifestations of binaural interference on behavioral and electrophysiological measures, and on some subjective complaints associated with the phenomenon. The first case was an older adult with a bilateral, symmetric sensorineural hearing loss who evidenced markedly asymmetric word-recognition scores under earphones in quiet. Word-recognition testing under the three conditions (aided right, aided left, and aided binaurally) in sound field revealed the binaurally aided score to be markedly poorer than the best monaurally aided score. This is the classic presentation of binaural interference. The second case was instructive in revealing an electrophysiological, as well as behavioral correlate of binaural interference. The auditory AMLR responses mirrored the speech-recognition findings; that is the Pa peak amplitude for binaural stimulation was markedly less than that for monaural stimulation of the better ear. In the last case of binaural interference, dichotic sentence testing was done in the free-report mode, which revealed markedly asymmetric scores, and in the directed-report mode, which should have resulted in improved performance in the poorly performing ear if attentional issues were the culprit in this 90-year-old individual. However, performance in the directed-report condition essentially was unchanged from that in the free-report condition. To rule out memory issues, the ear to be attended was precued and also post-cued, but the dichotic results remained unchanged by the cueing. To test the possibility that an age-related decline in the corpus callosum could explain the large interaural dichotic difference of 80–90%, the authors employed the P300 paradigm and found a P300 peak that was robust for the right ear, but greatly attenuated for the left ear for verbal targets. The reverse finding occurred for nonverbal material (right hemisphere would be dominant for non-verbal material in most individuals); the P300 peak was robust for the left ear and greatly attenuated for the right ear. The authors concluded that the best explanation for these findings was age-related changes in the corpus callosum.

In Chapter 5, we introduced screening and follow-up protocols for clinical assessment of binaural interference. These protocols are based on research findings to date, and should be revised as future research sheds further light on the phenomenon. The suggested arrangement for listener and loudspeakers is speech through the loudspeaker at 0° azimuth and competition through a separate loudspeaker at 180° azimuth (see Figure 5–1).

Screening Protocol

1. Perform behavioral speech-recognition testing (unaided mode) in sound field under the binaural (both ears open), monaural right ear (left ear plugged), and monaural left ear (right ear plugged) conditions.
2. Use speech materials that are based on the adaptive procedure with competition (e.g., speech babble) and are commercially available (e.g., HINT or QuickSIN). The outcome measure should be a signal-to-noise ratio (SNR).

Follow-Up Protocol if Screening Is Failed

1. The history should explore whether the chief complaint is suggestive of binaural interference (interaural differences, difficulty in noise, or other competitive listening situations, difficulties in the auditory spatial dimension, preference for one over two hearing aids). The history would be enhanced by the use of a questionnaire, such as the short form of the Speech, Spatial and Qualities of Hearing Scale (SSQ12), Noble et al. (2013).
2. A complete audiological evaluation should be performed, including performance-intensity functions for PB words (monaural right, monaural left, and binaural modes), static and dynamic acoustic-immittance assessment.
3. Repeat #1 in the screening protocol under the aided mode (binaurally aided, monaurally right aided, and monaurally

left aided), if the individual is aided or amplification is being considered. Given that binaural interference already has been identified during screening, testing under the monaurally aided mode need not involve plugging of the contralateral ear.

4. Employ physiological/electrophysiological tests to establish if electrophysiological correlates of binaural interference exist. The presence of such correlate(s) not only confirms the diagnosis of binaural interference, but also helps to establish the site(s) of interference.

In Chapter 6, we suggested that given the evolutionary advantage of two ears for directionality and space perception, which is critical for survival of animals in the wild, these auditory dimensions might be those most sensitive to alterations in binaural advantage and disadvantage. This principle underscores the importance of employing at least a two-loudspeaker arrangement as proposed in the clinical protocol. There is a need for future research testing arrangements in both aided and unaided conditions involving multiple loudspeakers, varying azimuths between speakers, and varying competing babble levels. Such test arrangements can yield directional error scores, as well as the standard outcome measure of correct speech recognition score. These are fruitful areas for future research.

Chapter 6 also notes the new avenue of research on binaural interference forged by Lina Reiss and her colleagues (2016, 2017), based on speculation that abnormal binaural spectral integration might explain the binaural interference observed on the vowel classification patterns of some individuals with hearing loss. This new avenue involves interaural pitch matching and dichotic fusion range measurement. Do individuals fuse sounds simultaneously presented to the two ears that are far apart versus close together in pitch?

References

Aboitiz, F., Rodriguez, E., Olivares, R., & Zaidel, E. (1996). Age-related changes in fibre composition of the human corpus callosum: Sex differences. *Neuroreport*, *7*, 1761–1764.

Allen, R., Schwab, B., Cranford, J., & Carpenter, M. (2000). Investigation of binaural interference in normal-hearing and hearing-impaired adults. *Journal of the American Acadamy of Audiology*, *11*, 494–500.

Arkebauer, H., Mencher, G., & McCall, C. (1971). Modification of speech discrimination in patients with binaural asymmetrical hearing loss. *Journal of Speech and Hearing Disorders*, *36*, 208–212.

Bellis, T. (2002). *When the brain can't hear* (pp. 135–161). New York, NY: Pocket Books.

Bellis, T., Nicol, T., & Kraus, N. (2000). Aging affects hemispheric asymmetry in the neural representation of speech sounds. *Journal of Neuroscience*, *20*, 791–797.

Bellis, T., & Wilber, L. (2001). Effects of aging and gender on interhemispheric function. *Journal of Speech, Language, and Hearing Research*, *44*, 246–263.

Bocca, E., Calearo, C., Cassinari, V., & Migliavacca, F. (1955). Testing "cortical" hearing in temporal lobe tumours. *Acta Otolaryngologica*, *45*, 289–304.

Boothroyd, A. (1993). Recovery of speech perception performance after prolonged auditory deprivation. *Journal of the American Academy of Audiology*, *4*, 331–336.

Boymans, M., Goverts, S., Kramer, S., Festen, J., & Dreschler, W. (2009). Candidacy for bilateral hearing aids: A retrospective multicenter study. *Journal of Speech, Language, and Hearing Research*, *52*, 130–140.

Bozgeyik, Z., Burakgazi, G., Sen, Y., & Ogur, E. (2008). Age-related metabolic changes in the corpus callosum: Assessment with MRI spectroscopy. *Diagnostic and Interventional Radiology*, *14*, 173–176.

Brooks, D., & Bulmer, D. (1981). Survey of binaural hearing aid users. *Ear and Hearing*, *2*, 220–224.

Bryden, M., Munhall, K., & Allard, F. (1983). Attentional biases and the right-ear effect in dichotic listening. *Brain and Language, 18,* 236–248.

Carter, A., Noe, C., & Wilson, R. (2001). Listeners who prefer monaural to binaural hearing aids. *Journal of the American Academy of Audiology, 12,* 261–272.

Chmiel, R., Jerger, J., Murphy, E., Pirozzolo, F., & Tooley-Young, C. (1997). Unsuccessful use of binaural amplification by an elderly person. *Journal of the American Academy of Audiology, 8,* 1–10.

Chung, S., & Stephens, S. (1986). Factors influencing binaural hearing aid use. *British Journal of Audiology, 20,* 129–140.

Cox, R., Schwartz, K., Noe, C., & Alexander, G. (2011). Preference for one or two hearing aids among adult patients. *Ear and Hearing, 32,* 181–197.

Day, G., Browning, G., & Gatehouse, S. (1988). Benefit from binaural hearing aids in individuals with severe hearing impairment. *British Journal of Audiology, 22,* 273–277.

Dillon, H., Birtles, G., & Lovegrove, R. (1999). Measuring the outcomes of a national rehabilitation program: Normative data for the Client Oriented Scale of Improvement (COSI) and the Hearing Aid Users Questionnaire (HAUQ). *Journal of the American Academy of Audiology, 10,* 67–79.

Edgington, E. (1967). Statistical inference from N=1 experiments. *Journal of Psychology, 65,* 195–199.

Erdman, S., & Sedge, R. (1981). Subjective comparisons of binaural versus monaural amplification. *Ear and Hearing, 2,* 225–229.

Gazzaniga, M., Ivry, R., & Mangun, G. (2002). *Cognitive neuroscience: The biology of the mind.* New York, NY: Norton.

Harford, E., & Dodds, E. (1966). The clinical application of CROS: A hearing aid for unilateral deafness. *Archives of Otolaryngology, 83,* 455–464.

Henkin, Y., Waldman, A., & Kishon-Rabin, L. (2007). The benefits of binaural versus unilateral amplification for the elderly: Are two always better than one? *Journal of Basic and Clinical Physiology and Pharmacology, 18,* 201–216.

Hill, J., & Purdy, S. (2011). Predictors of bilateral hearing aid success in older adults with hearing impairment. *Bulletin of the New Zealand Audiological Society, 21,* 17–51.

Holmes, A. (2003). Bilateral amplification for the elderly: Are two aids better than one? *International Journal of Audiology, 42*(Suppl. 2), 2S63–2S67.

Hurley, R. (1993). Monaural ear effect: Case presentations. *Journal of theAmerican Academy of Audiology, 4,* 285–295.

Jacobson, J., McCandless, G., & Mahoney, T. (1979). Influence of amplification on the discrimination of dichotic consonant-vowel syllables in a population with sensorineural hearing loss. *Audiology, 18,* 522–536.

Jerger, J., Alford, B., Lew, H., Rivera, V., & Chmiel, R. (1995). Dichotic listening, event-related potentials, and interhemispheric transfer in the elderly. *Ear and Hearing, 16,* 482–498.

Jerger, J., Chmiel, R., Allen, J., & Wilson, A. (1994). Effects of age and gender on dichotic sentence identification. *Ear and Hearing, 15,* 274–286.

Jerger, J., Darling, R., & Florin, E. (1994). Efficacy of the cued listening task in the evaluation of binaural hearing aids. *Journal of the American Academy of Audiology, 5,* 279–285.

Jerger, J., & Jordan, C. (1992). Age-related asymmetry on a cued-listening task. *Ear and Hearing, 13,* 272–277.

Jerger, J., Silman, S., Lew, H., & Chmiel, R. (1993). Case studies in binaural interference: Converging evidence from behavioral and electrophysiological measures. *Journal of the American Academy of Audiology, 4,* 122–131.

Jerger, J., Silman, S., Silverman, C., & Emmer, M. (2017). Binaural interference: Quo vadis? *Journal of the American Academy of Audiology, 29,* 266–270.

Jerger, J., Stach, B., Johnson, K., Loiselle, L., & Jerger, S. (1990). Patterns of abnormality in dichotic listening in the elderly. In

J. Jensen (Ed.), *Presbyacusis and other age-related aspects: 14th annual Danavox Symposium* (pp. 143–150). Copenhagen, Denmark: Danavox.

Karsten, S., & Turner, C. (2000). Binaural speech recognition and the Stenger effect. *Journal of Speech, Language, and Hearing Research, 43*, 926–933.

Kimura, D. (1961). Cerebral dominance and the perception of verbal stimuli. *Canadian Journal of Psychology, 15*, 166–171.

Knudsen, V. (1939). An ear to the future. *Journal of the Acoustical Society of America, 11*, 29–36.

Köbler, S., Lindblad, A., Olofsson, A., & Hagerman, B. (2010). Successful and unsuccessful users of bilateral amplification: Differences and similarities in binaural performance. *International Journal of Audiology, 49*, 613–627.

Lazard, D., Collette, J., & Perrot, X. (2011). Speech processing: From peripheral to hemispheric asymmetry of the auditory system. *Laryngoscope, 122*, 167–173.

Leek, M. (2001). Adaptive procedures in psychophysical research. *Perception and Psychophysics, 63*, 1279–1292.

Leigh-Paffenroth, E., Roup, C., & Noe, C. (2011). Behavioral and electrophsiologic binaural processing in persons with symmetric hearing loss. *Journal of the American Academy of Audiology, 22*, 181–193.

Levitt, H. (1971). Transformed up-down methods in psychoacoustics. *Journal of the Acoustical Society of America, 49*, (Suppl. 2), 467–477.

McArdle, R., Killion, M., Mennite, M., & Chisolm, T. (2012). Are two ears not better than one? *Journal of the American Academy of Audiology*, *23*, 171–181.

Møller, A. (2000). *Hearing: Its physiology and pathophysiology*. San Diego, CA: Academic Press.

Mussoi, B., & Bentler, R. (2017). Binaural interference and the effects of age and hearing loss. *Journal of the American Academy of Audiology, 28*, 5–13.

Neuman, A. (2005). Central auditory system plasticity and aural rehabilitation of adults. *Journal of Rehabilitation Research and Development, 42,* (Suppl. 2), 169–186.

Noble, W., Jensen, S., Naylor, G., Bhullar, N., & Akeroyd, M. (2013). A short form of the Speech, Spatial and Qualities of Hearing scale suitable for clinical use: The SSQ12. *International Journal of Audiology, 52,* 409–412.

Oh, Y., & Reiss, L. (2017). Binaural pitch fusion: Pitch averaging and dominance in hearing-impaired listeners with broad fusion. *Journal of the Acoustical Society of America, 142,* 780–791.

Picton, T. (2011). *Human auditory evoked potentials.* San Diego, CA: Plural.

Reiss, L., Eggleston, J., Walker, E., & Oh, Y. (2016). Two ears are not always better than one: Mandatory vowel fusion across spectrally mismatched ears in hearing-impaired listeners. *Journal of the Association for Research in Otolaryngology, 17,* 341–356.

Reiss, L., Shayman, C., Walker, E., Bennet, E., Fowler, J., Hartling, C., Glickman, B., . . . Oh, Y. (2017). Binaural pitch fusion: Comparison of normal-hearing and hearing-impaired listeners. *Journal of the Acoustical Society of America, 141,* 1909–1920.

Rothpletz, A., Tharpe, A., & Grantham, D. (2004). The effect of asymmetrical signal degradation on binaural speech recognition in children and adults. *Journal of Speech, Language, and Hearing Research, 47,* 269–280.

Schoepflin, J. (2007). Binaural interference in a child: A case study. *Journal of the American Academy of Audiology, 18,* 515–521.

Schreurs, K., & Olsen, W. (1985). Comparison of monaural and binaural hearing aid use on a trial period basis. *Ear and Hearing, 6,* 198–202.

Silman, S. (1995). Binaural interference in multiple sclerosis: Case study. *Journal of the American Academy of Audiology, 6,* 193–196.

Silman, S., Gelfand, S., & Silverman, C. (1984). Late-onset auditory deprivation: Effects of monaural versus binaural hearing aids. *Journal of the Acoustical Society of America, 76,* 1357–1362.

Silman, S., Jerger, J., Fanning, R., Silverman, C., & Emmer, M. (1998). Asymmetric suprathreshold speech recognition and the telephone ear phenomenon. *Journal of the American Academy of Audiology, 9*, 380–384.

Silverman, C., & Emmer, M. (1993). Auditory deprivation and recovery in adults with asymmetric sensorineural hearing impairment. *Journal of the American Academy of Audiology, 4*, 338–346.

Silverman, C., & Silman, S. (1990). Apparent auditory deprivation from monaural amplification and recovery with binaural amplification: Two case studies. *Journal of the American Academy of Audiology, 1*, 175–180.

Stephens, S., Callaghan, D., Hogan, S. Meredith, R., Rayment, A., & Davis, A. (1991). Acceptability of binaural hearing aids: A crossover study. *Journal of the Royal Society of Medicine, 84*, 267–269.

Stubblefield, J., & Nye, C. (1989). Aided and unaided time-related differences in word discrimination. *Hearing Instruments, 40*, 38–43.

Takeda, S., Yamada, S., Ono, S., & Matsuzawa, T. (1988). Age-related changes in the size of the corpus callosum: Magnetic resonance imaging. *Japanese Journal of Geriatrics, 25*, 292–295.

Thornton, A., & Raffin, M. (1978). Speech discrimination scores modeled as a binomial variable. *Journal of Speech and Hearing Research, 21*, 507–518.

Vaughan-Jones, R., Padgham, N., Christmas, H., & Irwin J. (1993). One aid or two?—More visits please! *Journal of Laryngology and Otology, 107*, 329–332.

Walden, T., & Walden, B. (2005). Unilateral versus bilateral amplification for adults with impaired hearing. *Journal of the American Academy of Audiology, 16*, 574–584.

Watson, L., & Tolan, T. (1949). *Hearing tests and hearing instruments*. Baltimore, MD: Williams and Wilkins.

Wieselberg, M., & Iório, M. (2012). Hearing aid fitting and unilateral auditory deprivation: Behavioral and electrophysiologic assessment. *Brazilian Journal of Otorhinolaryngology, 78*, 69–76.

Xiong, Y., & Mok, V. (2011). Age-related white matter changes. *Journal of Aging Research*. https://doi.org/10.4061/2011/617927

Index

Note: Page numbers in **bold** reference non-text material.

A

I

J

K

L

M

N

O

T